Nutrition   Health

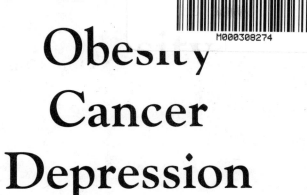

Obesity
Cancer
Depression

Their Common Cause & Natural Cure

You are not sick, you are thirsty!
Regain your vibrant health with water

F. Batmanghelidj, M.D.

Author of
Your Body's Many Cries for Water

A Healer's Guide to Natural Health
www.watercure.com

Obesity, Cancer, Depression
Their Common Cause and Natural Cure

Copyright © 2004 Fereydoon Batmanghelidj, M.D.
ISBN 0-9702458-2-3

First Edition: April 2005

Global Health Solutions, Inc.
2146 King's Garden Way
Falls Church, VA 22043
Telephone: 703-848-2333
Fax: 703-848-0028
Web site: www.watercure.com

To Our
Creator:
In Awe
with Humility
Dedication
and
Love

WATER CURE

"One man's solution to soaring health costs: water."
Paul Harvey

"Thanks to Dr. Batmanghelidj. I put your book next to the Bible and I read them both."
Dick Gregory

"Thanks again. You have truly made the world a better place."
Amazon.com Reviews

"The Greatest Single Discovery In The History Of The World."
Trevor James Constable
Author, Historian, Lecturer, Scientist
Borderlands **Quarterly** *Journal of Borderland Research*

"The water principle has a convincing logic but turns much of current medical practice on its head. Does it work? You only have to turn on the tap to find out."
The European, **London, December 1995**

"He is arguing for a new scientific approach that turns clinical medicine on its head."
The Daily Telegraph, **London, England**

"I was particularly stunned by Dr. Batmanghelidj's lucid description of how lack of water is the primary cause of hypertension, which affects 50 million Americans."
Julian Whitaker, M.D., *Health & Healing*

"It is claimed that fish probably have no awareness of the presence of water; this book shows we may have done little better.
Mostly we have treated symptoms, and often wrongly at that, but
masterpieces come into being to produce paradigm shifts. If we
learn this one, we may arrest the course of our patients in their
all too rapid going the way of all flesh."
Book Reviews, *Journal of Clinical Gastroenterology*

"The Greatest Health Discovery in the World."
Sam Biser, *The University of Natural Healing*

"After having read many of Dr. Batmanghelidj's recent works,
including his jewel of a book, Your Body's Many Cries for Water,
it is very apparent that this work is revolutionary and sweeps
nearly all diseases before it. As an Internist/Cardiologist I find
this work incisive, trenchant and fundamental. This work is a
God Send for all."
Dan C. Roehm, M.D., F.A.C.P.

"How like 'monkey mind' to bounce about, tying itself in knots
with complex solutions while ignoring the profound significance
of the simple! Circumstance helped Dr. Batmanghelidj perceive
the elegant significance of one factor we too often overlook:
water."
Jule Klotter, *Townsend Letter for Doctors*

"Dr. Batmanghelidj has researched the phenomenon of pain and
water metabolism of the body. His research, published in various
scientific journals, has led him to address pain as "proven but seldom recognized signal of local shortage of water in the body."
The Rotarian

Doctor Finds Ulcer Remedy
"It started with a patient suffering unbearable ulcer pain one late night. The Doctor treated him with 500 cubic centimeter of water. His pain became less severe and then disappeared completely. The physician was so impressed that he prescribed two glasses of water six times a day and achieved a "clinical" cure of the ulcer attack."
The New York Times "Science Watch"

"When Dr. Batmanghelidj thinks of a glass of water, he doesn't think of it as half full or half empty. He thinks of it as brimming over with the essential fluid of life. He thinks of it as the solvent of our ills and the deliverer of ripe old age. He thinks of it as the wave of the future."
The Washington Times

A Medical Atom Bomb!
"New! This book by a highly respected M.D. explodes a medical atom bomb--An entirely new paradigm for the cause and prevention of many degenerative diseases! You owe it to yourself to read this incredible book!"
Nutri-Books

"The average American is woefully uninformed about water. Most people think they drink enough water, but they don't. Dr. Batmanghelidj's book will create a tide of public opinion about the wonders of water."
The Connection Newspaper

"We have, he says in a new and highly controversial book, Your Body's Many Cries for Water, forgotten how to respond to our numerous thirst signals. But if, instead of taking painkillers and medication, we just drank lots of ordinary tap water, we would probably find that not only the pain, but also the condition would go away for ever."
The Independent, London, England

"Stomach pains, migraines, allergies, asthma, and even arthritis may all be symptoms of dehydration that could easily be cured by a few more glasses of household tap water. But only drinking water when you are feeling thirsty will not provide you with enough, according to F. Batmanghelidj, whose controversial book, *Your Body's Many Cries for Water*, sold tens of thousands of copies in the United States last year. "
Daily Mail, London, England

"Dr. Batman's books are full of common sense and truthful medical advice. His suggested treatment of diseases goes to the roots, the cause of it and anyone who is fortunate enough to read them won't be disappointed with their purchase."
**Laurence A. Malone, M.D., Ph.D., Dean for Academic Affairs,
The Learning Center for College Sciences, Ohio**

"I consider your insights some of the most amazing I have encountered in medicine. Sixteen years of private practice in OBG and 8 years as a GP have provided me with a perspective that appreciates the potentials of your proposals."
L. B. Works, M.D., F.A.G.C.O.

"The author, as a result of his extensive clinical and scientific research, concludes that the body possesses many different thirst signals. Many different symptoms and signs of dehydration have until now been viewed as classical diseases of the body."
**Frontier Perspectives,
The Center for Frontier Sciences at Temple University**

"After many years of study and practicing medicine, it is both rewarding and refreshing to discover the solution to many degenerative conditions beautifully explained by Dr. Batmanghelidj in *Your Body's Many Cries for Water*. This type of information fills a void left from traditional education."
Robert Battle, M.D.

"Thank you for the timely advice on using the combination of water and salt to treat my asthma... not only calmed my coughing but took it away. Once again thank you so much for sharing such insights into complex problems."
Jose A. Rivera, M.D.

"It is a well written book and easy to understand. I think reading of this book should be made compulsory in all the Elementary, Middle and High Schools. It will prevent lots of illnesses and suffering at almost no additional costs."
Hiten Shah, M.D.,
San Jacinto Medical Clinic, CA.

"Batmanghelidj leads us through these entities point by point and weaves a magnificent tapestry if not possibly allopathic medicine's shroud--we can't both be right."
The Biotron Connection

"Batmanghelidj's book, Your Body's Many Cries for Water, hits the nail on the head-period."
Arthur Moll, D.C.

Small Press Selection:
"Your Body's Many Cries for Water, a health book authored by a doctor combining holistic and medical facts about the effects of water and its healing possibilities on many diseases. This book was chosen since water is a topic that has increasing awareness in the marketplace and the author has credentials."
Jan Nathan, Executive Director,
Publishers Marketing Association

"Both these books, as well as the publishing firm, bring the sort of news that could change your life. Claims and counter-claims aside, Dr. Batmanghelidj has really got hold of something."
The Book Reader

"No pills! No pain! No fooling! ARTHRITIS CURE IN YOUR KITCHEN. Doctor's discovery heals for pennies a day."
National Examiner, December 14, 1993

"Yours is the most elegant description of arthritic pain I've ever read!"
Perry A. Chapdelaine, Sr., M.A.
Executive Director,
The Arthritis Fund/The Rheumatoid Disease Foundation

"Dynamite! Your hypothesis is precisely the paradigm breakthrough that generates quantum leaps forward in disease etiology."
Edmund H. Handwerger, D.D.S., M.P.H.

"Batmanghelidj gives example of patients who have followed his advice using ordinary tap water with positive results in reduction of blood pressure, allergy relief and weight loss. He even goes so far as to link the lack of water with depression."
The Irish Times

"It does seem sensible to adhere to the logic of the natural and the simple in medicine as fostered in the book, Your Body's Many Cries for Water."
Monsignor Philip A. Gray

"The content of your book is a huge gulp of fresh air, and holds much hope for the human race!"
Judge John B. Morgan, California

"I consider Dr. Batman's information as God-sent. It is my prayer that you too will benefit from his pain-relieving and life-extension revelations."
Lloyd Palmer, Straws in the Wind Newsletter, February 1996

"He has successfully treated allergies, angina, asthma, arthritis, headaches, hypertension, ulcers and more with the simplest of solutions-- water."
Nexus Magazine, Australia, January 1996

"As his controversial book quietly gathers support worldwide, the doctor behind one of medicine's most extraordinary theories explains why he has turned his back on conventional wisdom to treat his patients with water, not drugs"
Daily Mail, UK, August 27, 2001

"Revolutionary medical breakthrough: The slimming new water cure! Learn how to drink away 40 lbs."
Finola Hughes
All my Children TV series
Woman's World (cover)
September 4, 2001

"Dr. Batmanghelidj's discovery regarding water was critical to my recovery. I could not have recovered without it."
Lorraine Day, M.D.
Positive Press
Interview with Bob Butts

ACKNOWLEDGMENT AND GRATITUDE

My gratitude goes to two eminent cancer researchers of our times, Dr. M. Jawed Iqbal and Dr. John G. Delinassios, for their parts in introducing my views on the paradigm shift in medical science to other eminent cancer researchers in 1987 and in having my guest lecture at their conference published for future reference:

M. Jawed Iqbal, Ph.D., was the research director and head of the Tumor Biology Unit of the Department of Surgery at Kings College School of Medicine and Dentistry of London University in 1986 when he first became aware of my findings that dehydration is the primary cause of pain and disease, including cancer, in the human body. He was asked by the Foundation for the Simple in Medicine to evaluate my thesis that chronic unintentional dehydration is the cause of cancer formation in the human body. In the tradition of all past chemists, he spent six months trying to discover what element becomes the active agent that causes cancer. When he could find no particular element that could possibly trigger cancer cell formation, he was upset at his wasted time. I pointed out to him that when the body gets chronically and increasingly dehydrated, it suffers a multisystem upheaval in its regulatory physiological functions—to the point that cancer could result, because all the checks and balances in body chemistry disintegrate.

His own words describe what happened next: "Suddenly, I became aware of a totally new horizon to research. A subsequent six months' evaluation of the systems approach to disease made a four-dimensional view to disease emergence possible. All of a sudden, the foundation's systems approach, as a grassroots basis for future research, made absolute sense—at the same time that it exposed the insufficiency of the solutes approach to the art of the soluble."

John G. Delinassios, Ph.D., is the founder of the International Institute of Cancer Research in Greece and the editor in chief of the internationally acclaimed journal Anticancer Research. Dr. Iqbal and Dr. Delinassios got together and agreed to convene an international workshop of cancer researchers to hear and discuss my physiological approach to cancer formation in the body. This conference took place October 15–18, 1987, in Chalkis, Greece. My guest lecture, "Pain: A Need for Paradigm Change," was published in *Anticancer Research: International Journal of Cancer Research and Treatment*, Vol. 7, no. 5B (Sept.–Oct. 1987).

Among the eminent cancer researchers who became aware of the value of systems approach to future cancer research, and recognized its merit, was Professor G. P. Murphy, then director of Cancer Research Society.

Alas, if the use of water for cancer prevention had commercial value, it would have been a thoroughly researched process by now, and this book—the only published information on chronic unintentional dehydration and cancer formation in the body—would have been redundant.

F. Batmanghelidj, M.D

October 2004

Author's Note

The information and recommendations on water intake presented in this book are based on my training, personal experience, very extensive research, and other publications on the topic of water metabolism of the body. I do not dispense medical advice or prescribe the use or the discontinuance of any medication as a form of treatment without the advice of an attending physician, either directly or indirectly. My intent, based on the most recent knowledge of micro-anatomy and molecular physiology, is to offer information on the importance of water to well-being, and to help inform the public and medical professionals of the damaging effects of chronic unintentional dehydration to the body, from childhood to old age.

This book is not intended as a replacement for sound medical advice from a physician. On the contrary, sharing of the information contained in this book with the attending physician is highly desirable. Application of the information and recommendations described herein are undertaken at the individual's own risk. The adoption of the information should be in strict compliance with the instructions given herein. Very sick persons with a past history of major diseases and who are under professional supervision, particularly those with severe renal disease, should not make use of the information contained herein without the supervision of their attending physician.

This book is intended to open your eyes to new possibilities that would ultimately emancipate societies throughout the world from the dark ages of medicine established on the foundations of scientific ignorance of the human body, and the fraud of those who preserve the status quo and make money in the process. You are urged to read more on the topic before you begin to apply the information to your own personal health problems. This request is intended to protect you against jumping to conclusions without recognizing their ramifications.

All the recommendations and procedures herein contained are made without guarantee on the part of the author or the publisher, their agents, or employees. The author and publisher disclaim all liability in connection with the use of the information presented herein.

CONTENTS

Author's Note

Preface

Must-Read Letter and Article on Waiting to Get Thirsty

PART 1: OBESITY

PART 2: DEPRESSION

PART 3: CANCER

PREFACE

As a 73-year-old medical doctor, I am ashamed of the way we have let the drug industry highjack our once honorable profession and take control of our pens to sell their chemicals, which obviously hurt and kill people. I will provide proof of this in the pages that follow. Here, I would like to air my grievances with some professors and academicians who exercise silence when their obviously mistaken pronouncements are brought to their attention. When their statements are put under a magnifying glass, it becomes clear that the intension is to protect the status quo in medicine, where the drug industry is the ruthless king.

My conscience does not let me keep quiet. When I came to America in 1982, I arrived with the hope that my breakthrough discovery about the pain-relieving properties of water would be picked up by some teaching institution and, upon its verification, would make a positive difference in the lives of the people of the world. I was sadly mistaken. That did not happen, but I did not stop. To further my research, the Foundation for the Simple in Medicine was formed by a personal friend. Further research revealed where medicine of the 20th century had gone wrong—to the extent that manifestations of dehydration had been viewed as if they were diseases of unknown cause. They were, and they still are, treated with toxic chemicals—when all that the body needs is to have its thirst quenched!

Alas, neither the National Institutes of Health, the American Medical Association, nor the Department of Health and Human Services was interested. In fact, the NIH managed to censor my presentation on the neurotransmitter histamine as the body's primary water regulator and remove it from the report of the first Alternative Medicine Conference in Chantilly, Virginia, September 14–16, 1992. The NIH also stopped the National Library of

Medicine from indexing the articles that were published by the foundation. Even this did not stop me. I formed Global Health Solutions and took my findings in the form of books and tapes directly to the public. Through the medium of talk radio I started educating the public about the importance of proper hydration and not waiting to get thirsty in order to top up the body with water.

In less than 10 years, sales of bottled water surged, and most people seemed to be carrying a bottle of water when they were on the move. This change in the water-drinking habits of younger Americans must have alarmed the sick-care system in this country, which thrives on people remaining thirsty and being medicated to early death. Something that I consider a crime was done to stop people from drinking water to prevent thirst. It could not have been the soda makers behind it, because the "big boys" in this industry make more money out of bottled water than they do from soda.

Out of nowhere reports of an article in the Journal of Physiology by Professor Heinz Valtin of Dartmouth College appeared in prominent newspapers and national television programs as if it were a great breakthrough in medicine that would save the lives of millions. The article told people that they should wait and only drink water when they get thirsty. Such an unusually disseminated directive could only be aimed at reestablishing the past, and scientifically asinine, view of thirst—a view that would save the future of the sick-care system and make the business of medicine expand and grow once again, at the expense of society's health and hard-earned wealth.

I could not bear seeing my many years of research on pain and water rendered ineffective by the orchestrated spread of the erroneous and harmful views of Dr. Valtin, recommending that people should wait until they get thirsty before they drink water—the very thing they were doing in the past that caused the monster medial quagmire we are in now. I wrote a scientific rebuttal to the good doctor's article and sent it to the editor of the physiology journal that had published his article. I even spoke with him in Berlin where he was teaching. He was most unenthusiastic to publish my rebuttal. After going the round of papers and journals to warn the public not to wait until they get thirsty, the Townsend Letters for Doctors and Patients, the Rolls-Royce of alternative medicine publications, published the article in its January 2003 issue.

The published article was now sent to most newspapers that had projected Dr. Valtin's views into the mind of the public. Not one of them wanted to touch the information; they obviously did not want to rock the boat of the commercial drug pushers. The actual article was posted on the Web site www.watercure.com for people to read and judge its validity for themselves; I am also including it at the end of this preface.I thought there should be a limit to the fraud of treating thirsty people with medications that sicken and prematurely kill them. The practice of medicine needs to once again reconstruct itself on its earlier foundations of integrity, empathy, and honesty.

You now have an idea of the odds that are stacked against the American people immediately benefiting from my brand of truth in medicine—*You Are Not Sick, You Are Thirsty*, what this book is all about. The media will do with this book what they did with the others: They will not promote it lest they lose income from the advertising dollars of the drug industry.

Must-Read Letter and Article on Waiting to Get Thirsty

LETTER TO DR. LAWRENCE APPEL:

back to the letters page

Professor Lawrence Appel, M.D., M.P.H.

Chairman: Food and Nutrition Panel
National Academy of Sciences, 26 February, 2004

Dear Dr. Appel:

Follow Your Thirst, Report Says: Washington Post
Thursday, February 12, 2004

Wrong! A large percentage of people get sick as a result of chronic unintentional dehydration without sensing thirst!

The view presented by your NAS panel about waiting to get thirsty before drinking water is exactly what is wrong with medicine in America, and possibly the single cause of escalating costs of the "sick care" system in this country. This is the reason we have a sick care system in place of having a health care system that understands disease prevention instead of medicating people until they get sicker by the millions. At least 200,000 of these die every year from medication-related problems. This is the very reason that after heart disease and cancer, chemicals used in patient treatment are the third most prevalent licensed and protected cause of death in this country, more than the other common diseases.

None of the honorable members of your panel, whose report made news in all the major media, seemed to be aware that PA Phillips, PA. and associates, New England J. Medicine, Sept. 1985—Reduced Thirst Water Deprivation in Healthy Elderly Men—have shown that sharpness of the perception of thirst is lost after a certain age until obviously dehydrated elderly do not recognize they need to drink water and do not reach for water that is put next to them. Otherwise your panel would have used different wording in their report. The elderly are the sickest sector of society as a result of waiting to get thirsty before they drink water, exactly what your report is recommending people should do.

Worse still, the panel seems to be unaware of the primary role of the neurotransmitter histamine as the water regulator and the drought management program coordinator in the body: that it gets more and more manufactured as the body begins to get dehydrated, producing the major localized pains and systemic conditions like allergies, asthma, the "inflammatory diseases," and others: that water is the best natural antihistamine that should be used instead of the antihistamine chemicals on the market: that water is the best natural diuretic that should be used in place of drugs for this purpose. With their drastic limitation of knowledge about the water regulatory processes in the human body, to dictate to people to drink water only when they get thirsty without doubt will harm most of those who trustingly heed the instruction. The abstract of presentation on histamine is attached.

Your panel has reiterated what Heinz Valtin, M.D., professor emeritus of Dartmouth Medical School, published in the American Journal of Physiology in August of 2002. My attached rebuttal article to Dr. Valtin's obsolete views about initiation of the thirst mechanism by the kidney—"Waiting to Get Thirsty Is to Die Prematurely and Very Painfully"—was published in the Townsend Letters for Doctors and Patients, January 2003. The article is also posted on www.watercure.com.

This article explains fully why the esteemed members of your panel need to review the published materials on unintentional dehydration and reverse the emphasis in their report on "waiting to get thirsty before drinking water"—as soon as possible. They need to realize that the body has many other emergency thirst signals that precede the dry mouth indicator of thirst. They need to advise people to minimally overhydrate—prevent dehydration—rather than wait for dehydration to cause a "dry mouth" before drinking water. A large percentage of people get sick as a result of locally settled and inflammation-producing chronic unintentional dehydration without sensing "thirst."

The members of your panel need to realize that water should be placed on top of the list of nutrients. After all, it is the primary instrument of energy release—its hydrolytic chemical action—for all functions in the human body. People who drink water to prevent thirst are doing the right thing. They are preventing the diseases of dehydration that we in medicine have assumed to be this or that disease condition and treated with inventive cocktails of toxic medications. This is the dark side of modern medicine that is getting exposed for the shameful, licensed and protected, medical ignorance that it is.

The enclosed books *Your Body's Many Cries for Water and Water Cures: Drugs Kill,* and my attached article—20th Century Medicine: The Product of 100 Years of Darkness—make the above points clear.

This letter will also be posted on our web site, and a copy will be sent to the editors of the Washington Post and some others who highlighted your report for the public to follow. People need to know the soundness of your panel's views on drinking water only when one gets "thirsty"—in the traditional sense of the word thirst expressed in the report—has been professionally, clinically, and scientifically challenged.

In the true tradition of academicians, I hope you will favor us with a few words of response so that it could be posted alongside this letter on our web site. Thank you.

Sincerely,
F. Batmanghelidj, M.D.
www.watercure.com

cc: Other members of Food and Nutrition Panel, NAS Editor, the Washington Post, LA Times, and others.

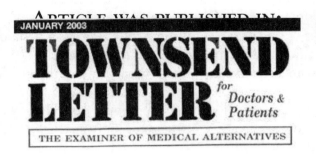

ARTICLE WAS PUBLISHED IN:

JANUARY 2003

TOWNSEND LETTER *for* Doctors & Patients

THE EXAMINER OF MEDICAL ALTERNATIVES

"Waiting to Get Thirsty Is to Die Prematurely and Very Painfully"

F. Batmanghelidj, M.D.

Heinz Valtin, M.D., an emeritus professor at Dartmouth Medical School, has ventured the opinion that there is no scientific merit in drinking 8 x 8-ounce glasses of water a day and not waiting to get thirsty before correcting dehydration. This view, published in the American Journal of Physiology, August 2002, is the very foundation of all that is wrong with modern medicine, which is costing this nation $1.7 trillion a year, rising at the rate of 12 percent every year. Dr. Valtin's view is as absurd as waiting for the final stages of a killer infection before giving the patient the appropriate antibiotics. His views are based on the erroneous assumption that dry mouth is an accurate sign of dehydration.

Like the colleagues he says he has consulted, Dr. Valtin does not seem to be aware of an important paradigm shift in medicine. All past views in medicine were based on the wrong assumption that it is the solutes in the body that regulate all functions and that the solvent has no direct role in any of the body's physiological functions. In medical schools it is taught that water is only a solvent, a packing material and a means of transport; that water has no metabolic function of its own. I have come across this level of ignorance about the primary physiological role of water at another Ivy League medical school from another eminent professor of physiology who, like

Dr. Valtin, researched and taught the water-regulatory mechanisms of the kidney to medical students and doctors. Only when I asked him what "hydrolysis" is did the penny drop and he admitted the scientific fact that water is a nutrient and does indeed possess a dominant metabolic role in all physiological functions of the body.

Dr. Valtin's emphasis on the water-regulatory role of the kidneys limits his knowledge to the body's mechanisms of "deficit management" of the water needs of the body. He seems to base his views of thirst management of the body on the vital roles of vasopressin, the antidiuretic hormone, and the renin-angiotensin system, the elements that get engaged in the drought-management programs of the body, when the body has already become dehydrated. Indeed, he thinks dehydration is a state of the body when it loses 5 percent of its water content; and that one should wait until at some level of such water loss the urge to drink some kind of "fluid" will correct the water deficit in the body. This view might have seemed plausible 25 years ago. Today, it exposes the tragic limitations of knowledge of the human physiology that is available to a prestigious medical school in America.

In his recently published and widely reported assertions, Dr. Valtin does not take into consideration the fact that water is a nutrient. Its vital "hydrolytic" role would be lost to all the physiological functions that would be affected by its shortage in its osmotically "free state." Another oversight is the fact that it is the interior of the cells of the body that would become drastically dehydrated. In dehydration, 66 percent of the water loss is from the interior of the cells, 26 percent of the loss is from extracellular fluid volume, and only 8 percent of the loss is borne by the blood tissue in the vascular system, which constricts within its network of capillaries and maintains the integrity of the circulation system.

Philippa M. Wiggin has shown that the mechanism that controls or brings about the effective function of the cation pumps utilizes the energy transforming property of water, the solvent; "The source of energy for cation transport or ATP synthesis lies in increases in chemical potentials with increasing hydration of small cations and polyphosphate anions in the highly structured interfacial aqueous phase of the two phosphorylated intermediates."[1] Waiting to get thirsty, when the body fluids become concentrated before thirst is induced, one loses the energy-generating properties of water in the dehydrated cells of the body. This is a major reason why we should prevent dehydration, rather than wait to correct it. This new understanding of the role of water in cation exchange is enough justification to let the body engage in prudent surplus water management rather than forcing it into drought and deficit water management, which is what Dr. Valtin is recommending people do.

In his research on the "conformational change in biological macromolecules," Ephraim Katchalski-Katzir of the Weizmann Institute of Science has shown that the "proteins and enzymes of the body function more efficiently in solutions of lower viscosity."[2] Thus, water loss from the interior of the cells would adversely affect their efficiency of function. This finding alone negates Dr. Valtin's view that we should let dehydration get established before drinking water. Since it is desirable that all cells of the body should function efficiently within their physiological roles, it would be more prudent to optimally hydrate the body rather than wait for the drought management programs of the body to induce thirst. Furthermore, it is much easier for the body to deal with a slight surplus of water than to suffer from its shortfall and have to ration and allocate water to vital organs at the expense of less vital functions of the body. The outcome of constantly circulating concentrated blood in the vascular system is truly an invitation to catastrophe.

The tragedy of waiting to get thirsty hits home when it is realized that the sharpness of thirst perception is gradually lost as we get older. Phillips and associates have shown that after 24 hours of water deprivation, the elderly still do not recognize they are thirsty: "The important finding is that despite their obvious physiologic need, the elderly subjects were not markedly thirsty."[3] Bruce and associates have shown that, between the ages of 20 and 70, the ratio of water inside the cells to the amount of water outside the cells drastically changes from 1.1 to 0.8.[4] Undoubtedly this marked change in the intracellular water balance would not take place if the osmotic push and pull of life could favor water diffusion through the cell membranes everywhere in the body—at the rate of 10^{-3} centimeters per second. Only by relying on the reverse osmotic process of expanding the extracellular water content of the body, so as to filter and inject "load-free" water into vital cells by the actions of vasopressin and the renin-angiotensin-aldosterone systems—when the body physiology is constantly forced to rely on its drought-management programs—could such a drastic change in the water balance of the body result.

Two other scientific discoveries are disregarded when Dr. Valtin recommends people should wait until they get thirsty before they drink water. One, the initiation of the thirst mechanisms is not triggered by vasopressin and the renin-angiotensin systems—these systems are only involved in water conservation and forced hydration of the cells. Thirst is initiated when the Na^+-K^+-ATPase pump is inadequately hydrated. It is water that generates voltage gradient by adequately hydrating the pump proteins in the neurotransmission systems of the body.[1] This is the reason the brain tissue is 85 percent water[5] and cannot endure the level of "thirst-inducing" dehydration that is considered safe in the article published by Dr. Valtin.

Two, the missing piece of the scientific puzzle in the water-regulatory mechanisms of the body, which has been exposed since 1987, and Dr. Valtin and his colleagues need to know about it, is the coupled activity of the neurotransmitter histamine to the efficiency of the cation exchange; its role in the initiation of the drought-management programs; and its role in the catabolic processes when the body is becoming more and more dehydrated.[5] Based on the primary water-regulatory functions of histamine, and the active role of water in all physiologic and metabolic functions of the body—as the hydrolytic initiator of all solute functions—the symptoms of thirst are those produced by excess histamine activity and its subordinate mechanisms, which get engaged in the drought-management programs of the body. They include asthma, allergies, and the major pains of the body, such as heartburn, colitis pain, rheumatoid joint pain, back pain, migraine headaches, fibromyalgic pains, and even anginal pain.[5, 6] And, since vasopressin and the renin-angiotensin-aldosterone activity in the body are subordinates to the activation of histamine, their role in raising the blood pressure is a part of the drought-management programs of the body.[6] Their purpose of forced delivery of water into vital cells demands a greater injection pressure to counteract the direction of osmotic pull of water from inside the cells of the body, when it is dehydrated.

From the new perspective of my 22 years of clinical and scientific research into molecular physiology of dehydration, and the peer-reviewed introduction of a paradigm shift in medical science, recognizing histamine as a neurotransmitter in charge of the water regulation of the body, I can safely say the 60 million Americans with hypertension, the 110 million with chronic pains, the 15 million with diabetes, the 17 million with asthma, the 50 million with allergies, and more, all did exactly as Dr. Valtin recommends. They all waited to get thirsty. Had they realized water is a natural antihistamine[5, 7, 8] and a more effective diuretic, these people would have been saved the agony of their health problems.

REFERENCES
1- Wiggins PM; A Mechanism of ATP-Driven Cation Pumps; PP-266-269, *Biophysics of Water*, Eds. Felix Franks and Sheila F. Mathis, John Wiley and Sons, Ltd., 1982

2- Ephraim Katchalski-Katzir: Conformational Changes In Biological Macromolecules; *Biorheology*, 21, PP. 57-74, 1984.

3- Phillips PA; Rolls BJ; Ledingham JGG; Forsling ML; Morton JJ; Crowe MJ and Wollner L; Reduced Thirst After Water Deprivation In Healthy Elderly Men; *The New England Journal of Medicine*, PP.753-759, Vol. 311, No. 12, Sept. 20 1985.

4- Bruce A, Anderson M, Arvidsson B, Isacksson B; Body Composition, Predictions of Normal Body Potassium, Body Water and Body Fat in Adults on the Basis of Body Height, Body Weight and Age; *Scand. J. Clin. Lab. Invest*, 40, 461-473, 1980.

5- Batmanghelidj F. M.D. Pain: A Need for Paradigm Change; *Anticancer Research*, Vol. 7, No. 5 B, PP. 971-990, Sept.- Oct. 1987; full article posted on www.watercure.com.

6- Batmanghelidj F. M.D.; *Your Body's Many Cries for Water*; Global Health Solutions, Inc.

7- Batmanghelidj F. M.D. Neurotransmitter Histamine: An Alternative View; Page 37 of the *Book of Abstracts*; The 3rd Interscience World Conference on Inflammation, Analgesics and Immunomodulators, Monte-Carlo, 1989. The Abstract and the full article are posted on the Web sitewww.watercure.com.

8- Batmanghelidj F M.D.; *ABC of Asthma, Allergies and Lupus*; Global Health Solutions, Inc.

I wrote this lengthy preface to share my concerns with you about the future of medicine in America. Unless you—yes, you, and people like you—get into the arena and demand the necessary changes in medicine, people in this country will remain cash cows to the drug industry. There is a limit to what people like me can do without your help. The ball is in your court.

I do hope Drs. Valtin and Appel—and the members of his Food and Nutrition Panel of the National Academy of Sciences—after reading the published materials I sent them, will revise and officially withdraw their views that people should wait to get thirsty before drinking water. By doing so, they would forever release humanity from the stranglehold of the drug industry. They should become aware that this view has already hurt a vast number of people. It has also made the drug industry more brazen in its presentation of falsehoods to sell drugs to people who are only manifesting one or another of the many symptoms and signs of unintentional dehydration, only because they waited to get thirsty. It is wrong that the national icons of science misguide people and then keep silent.

PART 1

OBESITY

CHAPTER 1

OBESITY
THE DIRECT CONSEQUENCE OF
UNINTENTIONAL DEHYDRATION

When I started my medical studies, if someone had told me that growing fat is the result of not drinking water, I would have said, Nonsense, have you gone mad? Today I would think twice before I reject the notion that not drinking water on a regular basis can result in excess fat deposits, to the point of causing deformity of the body. Bear with me while I explain the relationship of chronic unintentional dehydration to a gradual increase in the fat composition of the body, the initiating process in the development of a host of other health problems. Some might think it odd to address three disparate medical conditions in one book. You will be surprised to find what a close relationship there is between obesity and depression, and depression and cancer. Depressed people tend to overeat, and depression is the gateway to the development of cancer—hence their discussion together in this book.

To achieve my purpose of shedding light on obesity, cancer, and depression and their associated disease conditions, I will need to go back and explain the first principles of the science of physiology, their application to human metabolism, and the commanding role of the brain in all aspects of the individual's life.

I hope you will be patient so that, step by step, I can share with you the essence of my 24 years of research into the adverse effects of dehydration in the body, and its relationship to various health problems—in this case, obesity, depression, and cancer. I promise to make this book as readable and believable as I can, despite its many dips into complicated and traditionally jargon-riddled sci-

ence. I will also share with you some of the positive reports I have
received from people who suffered these health problems and
recovered using water and nutrition as natural guidelines.

Before we get into the main theme of this book, you need to understand the relationship of dehydration to not only gaining body
weight, but also all the attributed complications of obesity and the
vast array of human health problems, which are known to kill.
What you must grasp is the fact that the complications and deaths
traditionally blamed on obesity, depression, and cancer are actually
caused by persistent unintentional dehydration, the primary cause
of these defined disease states in the first place.

On Tuesday, May 5, 2003, the Science Times of the New York Times
reported extensively on an article, which was published in the New
England Journal of Medicine, on the relationship of various cancers
to excess weight. The researchers had followed 900,000 men and
women from 1982 to 1998, a 16-year linear study. They discovered
that the more overweight a person gets, the more there is the possi-
bility of developing cancer.

The preamble to the article states that while many may know that
excess pounds raise the risk of hypertension, heart disease, diabetes,
strokes, gallbladder disease, arthritis, and other debilitating and sometimes fatal health problems, now a host of cancers can be added to the
list. No longer is the list limited to cancers of the breast or uterus;
rather, cancers of colon, rectum, esophagus, pancreas, kidney, gallbladder, ovary, liver, and prostate, as well as multiple myeloma, lymphoma, and more, are linked to excess body weight. By the time you
finish this book, there will be no doubt in your mind about the relationship of obesity to dehydration. Since research has defined a relationship between cancer formation in the body and obesity, I am sure
you want to know how could dehydration cause cancer in the body.

The answer is simple. Dehydration causes a multifaceted disturbance
in the normal physiological functions in the body, which allows cancer to develop.

What the New York Times reported did not surprise me in the least. I explained this relationship in 1987 as the guest lecturer at an international cancer conference when I identified pain as a manifestation of dehydration that would lead to many diseases, including cancer. I will explain the physiology that allows cancer formation and disease production in the chapter on dehydration and cancer. The gist of this information was also the subject of my 2002 Cancer Control Society lecture—Dehydration and Cancer. The lecture was videotaped and is available for viewing.

WHY DO WE LET DEHYDRATION CAUSE DISEASE?

The answer is simple: Because the scientific foundation on which modern medicine is based has been structured around a number of false assumptions. Furthermore, until I came on the scene, no one had questioned these assumptions for the past 100 years of costly research into the diseases of the human body.

In the next few paragraphs, you will discover why we never understood dehydration. You will realize that you were not the only one who made this awful mistake; the medical and scientific communities, which spend your billions of dollars on their pet projects, were just as blind. All this time, we in medicine had labeled varying patterns of local or regional dehydration of the body as this or that disease. We invented our tongue-twisting jargon to label complications of water shortage in the body as a new discovery in medicine, and immediately asked for more money to expand on our labels.

What you will read in this book is the new foundation of thought in modern medicine, because I came to see the mistaken labeling through my own bitter experience. What I discovered is a medical breakthrough that will put the science of physiology in charge of the future of medicine. It will steer it away from the grip of the pharmaceutical industry and its malicious practice of using the sick in our society as cash cows. I have discovered the errors of basic scientific judgment on which the entire structure of modern medicine

has been constructed—in the process killing millions and making
tens of millions of people sicker because society thought we doctors
knew what we were doing. We hurt people, and the drug industry
made money from our blind ignorance of the way the human body
shows that it is short of water.

In case you take umbrage at this statement, proof of what I am saying can be found in the following headlines: Washington Post,
Wednesday, April 15, 1998 and November 21, 2003:

The Washington Post
WEDNESDAY, APRIL 15, 1998

Correctly Prescribed Drugs Take Heavy Toll

Millions Affected By Toxic Reactions

By RICK WEISS
Washington Post Staff Writer

More than 2 million Americans become seriously ill every year because of toxic reactions to correctly prescribed medicines taken properly, and 106,000 die from those reactions, a new study concludes. That surprisingly high number makes drug side effects at least the sixth, and perhaps even the fourth, most common cause of death in this country.

The Washington Post
FRIDAY, NOVEMBER 21, 2003

Reports from the Institute of Medicine, which is part of the congressionally chartered National Academy of Sciences, have no legal force but can be hugely influential. A report four years ago that estimated at least 44,000 Americans—and possibly as many as 98,000—die of medical errors each year riveted national attention on a subject that academic researchers had been trying to get the public to notice for years. The new report, called "Patient Safety: Achieving a New Standard of Care," was conceived as a first big step in solving the problems laid out in the earlier document, "To Err is Human."

If you add up the figures in the two articles, you will see that no less than 204,000 people die as a result of taking medications, and millions get sicker than before taking their prescribed drugs. These are very conservative estimates.

The irony of it all is that the drug industry knows its medications do not work in majority of cases. Here is the proof. The Independent is a prestigious British newspaper.

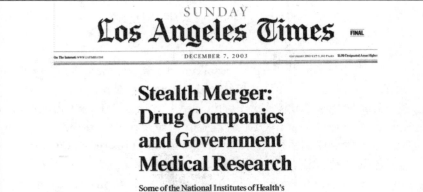

THE INDEPENDENT

Monday, December 8, 2003

Glaxo chief: Our drugs do not work on most patients

"The vast majority of drugs – more than 90 per cent – only work in 30 or 50 per cent of the people," Dr Roses said. "I wouldn't say that most drugs don't work. I would say most drugs work in 30 to 50 per cent of people. Drugs out there on the market work, but they don't work in everybody."

How do you think the drug companies can make billions of dollars from the sale of ineffective drugs? They buy their way into mainstream medical thought through the institutions of government.

SUNDAY

Los Angeles Times

FINAL

DECEMBER 7, 2003

Stealth Merger: Drug Companies and Government Medical Research

Some of the National Institutes of Health's top scientists are also collecting paychecks and stock options from biomedical firms. Increasingly, such deals are kept secret.

The shameful scientific assumptions—which have cost society dearly and have led people in the direction that they have become completely helpless and unwittingly get herded onto the doomsday train of the drug industry—are as follows:

FALSE ASSUMPTION NUMBER ONE:

*"Dry mouth is the only sign of
dehydration in the body."*

Actually, dry mouth is not a sign to rely on. The body can suffer from
deep dehydration inside its cells without manifesting a dry mouth symptom. You see, anytime you are short of water, 66 percent of the amount
is pulled out of the cells, 26 percent is taken from the environment
around the cells, and only 8 percent is lost from the blood. However, the
capillary bed begins to constrict and gradually shrink its wide network of
distribution to compensate for the water loss from blood circulation.
The big blood vessels are not affected. The blood composition is not
altered measurably enough that the deficiency becomes obvious. This is
why the body begins to suffer symptoms of drought in the interior of its
cells in the drought-stricken areas, while blood tests show nothing that
would explain the symptoms of localized drought.

Another mechanism that exists to prevent dry mouth is the way circulation to the salivary glands is increased to ensure ample saliva for chewing and swallowing food when the rest of the body begins to suffer from
water shortage.

Let me explain an important issue about dehydration. There are two
major classes of water in the body. One type of water is osmotically
engaged—it's already busy with some aspect of its different functions.
This class of water is not free to engage in new activity. Another type of
water is not osmotically engaged; it is free water. This type of water can
engage in new chemical reactions and important activities of the body
that need free water. For example, free water can get into the interior of
cells and correct water shortages before permanent damage can occur.
When I talk of dehydration, it really means the body is short of free
water to perform new water-dependent functions. For example, a 250-
pound diabetic has plenty of water in his tissues, but is short of free water
in the interior of his cells. The rise in the circulating blood's sugar level
is designed to not only prevent water from accompanying the sugar that
should rightly get into the cells, but also add to the osmotic pull of more

water out of the cells—hence intracellular dehydration, the killing process in diabetes.

The color of urine is a distinct marker of dehydration. When the urine is consistently very light to almost colorless, the body is blessed because it has ample supply of free water to get rid of its toxic waste without too much effort. When the urine becomes naturally and consistently yellow—not from pigments taken in the diet, such as vitamins, beet root, turmeric, and the like—it means the body is gradually getting short of its free water supply. The kidneys are working harder to get rid of the toxic waste from food metabolism. When the color of urine is consistently orange, it heralds serious health problems associated with severe dehydration. If the problems are not already apparent, trouble will reveal its ugly head sooner rather than later, perhaps in form of severe angina, strokes, or even sudden death from a massive heart attack.

The free water reserve of the body can only be maintained by its regular intake. The best form of free water is supplied when it is in its natural state. Manufactured beverages do not necessarily stay in the body long enough to perform the same functions as natural water. Most current additives to water in the manufacture of beverages are dehydrating agents.

Unfortunately, the power of advertising by the beverage industry, and the addictive nature of some of these beverages—in addition to the fact that the price structure grossly favors these soft drinks rather than water sold in convenient bottles—has captured the minds of the younger members of society. The outcome has been devastating. Young people are now getting fatter and fatter, and are developing all the disease complications of dehydration from their early preteens—60 percent of overweight children between 5 and 10 years of age have at least one of the risk factors for cardiovascular disease. We now see adult-onset diabetes and even hypertension among teenagers.

Dehydration in the interior of the cells produces severe symptoms, to the point of life-threatening crises, without the dry mouth of dehydration. Modern medicine has confused these symptoms of internal, localized droughts, identifying them as diseases. As a result, toxic medications are used until the person dies.

FALSE ASSUMPTION NUMBER TWO:

"Water is a simple inert substance that only dissolves,
circulates different things, and, ultimately, fills up the
empty spaces. It has no chemical role of its own in the
physiological functions of the body: All chemical actions
in the body are performed by the solid matter that are
dissolved in the water."

Water is not a simple inert substance. It is the single most complex element in nature. It is made up of two gases, oxygen and hydrogen, but assumes a liquid form. At 100 degrees Celsius it assumes a gaseous form. At 4 degrees Celsius it has the highest density; at 0 degrees, it becomes its lightest form. Why do you think it becomes so light? So that it can float on the surface of a body of water, permitting marine life to survive below. Otherwise—if rivers and lakes were to accumulate ice below their surfaces—nothing could survive a cold winter. You see, water is naturally designed to support life.

Water's functions in the body can be divided into two classes. First are its life-sustaining roles—its roles as a solvent, as a packing material that fills up all the spaces between the cells of the body, and as a transportation system in the bloodstream and the micro streams in the nerves and the muscles.

The other, more important role of water is its life-giving functions, or energy-generating actions. It manufactures hydroelectricity at the cell membranes: Its breakdown of food and its involvement in chemical reactions, known as hydrolysis, energizes all such functions. Perhaps most vital function are water's adhesive properties, which bond the solid structure of the cell membranes and protect life inside the cells of the body.

Modern medicine recognizes only the life-sustaining properties of water. This is why we never understood chronic unintentional dehydration as an ultimately deadly process. With a decreased intake of water, we gradually limit life processes in the body until a pattern of decay is established. This is why you need to recognize and understand the process that will naturally save your health and life. Don't expect the drug industry's medication to do it for you. All your body asks from you is timely intake of water. And don't let the jargon-peddlers in the drug industry force you to take expensive medications in place of the water your body is crying for.

FALSE ASSUMPTION NUMBER THREE:

*"The human body can regulate its water intake
efficiently throughout a person's life."*

This, too, is incorrect. As we grow older, we lose our perception of thirst and fail to drink adequately until the plum-like cells in vital organs become prune-like and can no longer sustain life. You need to recognize the onset of dehydration, and its manifestations, to prevent the irreversible stages of the process. The tragedy of waiting to get thirsty hits home when it is realized that as we get older, the sharpness of thirst perception is gradually lost.

Researchers Phillips and associates have shown that after 24 hours of water deprivation, the elderly still do not recognize they are thirsty: "The important finding is that despite their obvious physiologic need, the elderly subjects were not markedly thirsty." In other words, they did not recognize any thirst in their obviously dehydrated bodies.

Another group of researchers, Bruce and Associates, have shown that, between the ages of 20 and 70, the ratio of water inside the cells to the amount of water outside the cells drastically changes, from 1.1 to 0.8; meaning more water is around the cells than inside them—that by age 70, the plum-like cells are more prune-like. Undoubtedly, this marked symptom- and disease-producing change in the intracellular water balance would not take place if regular intake of water were maintained, allowing water to freely diffuse through the cell membranes everywhere in the body. Water usually diffuses through the cell membrane at an approximate rate of 0.03 centimeter per second. Very fast indeed, and only disengaged or "free water" can do this. Water that is already osmotically bound to other elements is unable to traverse through the cell membrane.

Only when the body physiology is constantly forced to rely on its drought-management programs could such a drastic change in the water balance between the inner cell and outer cell compartments of the body result. Plum-like cells become prune-like, and the normal physiology of the body is disrupted. We will discuss this issue more extensively later in the book.

FALSE ASSUMPTION NUMBER FOUR:

"Any fluid can meet the body's water needs:
All manufactured beverages and fluids will serve
the body in exactly the same way as water."

This is probably the most serious of all mistakes when it comes to fluid management of the body.

This mistake is background to all the health problems of our society at present. Through the power of advertising alone, the beverage industry has manipulated the lifestyle of everyone from toddlers to octogenarians.

Some of the manufactured beverages in common use today do not function in the body like natural water. If you begin to understand the natural reason some plants manufacture caffeine, or even cocaine, you will then recognize the problem. Even milk and fruit juices cannot meet the body's daily water needs. Like it or not, you have to get used to the taste of water: brand-name or even tap water. It is critical that you prevent thirst and dehydration regularly, and not wait to reach the kind of water that you perceive as tastier.

CHAPTER 2

WHY NOT OTHER BEVERAGES?

ALCOHOLIC BEVERAGES

- Alcohol disrupts the emergency water supply system to the brain. This causes brain dehydration, which presents itself as a hangover headache.

- Alcohol is addictive and functionally depressive.
  It dislocates the personality from the norms of behavior and creates social outcast.

- Alcohol causes impotence.

- Alcohol causes liver damage.

- Alcohol suppresses the immune system.

- Alcohol consumption increases the chances of developing cancers.

- Alcohol produces free radicals (acid-like substances) that normally attack and damage some sensitive tissues if allowed to circulate freely.

Among other things, melatonin is used up to scavenge these free radicals. This results in low melatonin content in the body. Alcohol shuts down the process that filters and injects water into most vital cells of the body when dehydration has established and water in its free state is not adequately available to seep into the cell through its membranes. The water injection process is known as reverse osmosis. In dehydration, water is pulled out of the cells and circulated in the bloodstream. In dehydration, the osmotic force of the blood is stronger than the osmotic force of the interior of the cells. The reason is simple. Potassium that holds on to the water inside the cells leaks out, and water will follow it. This same water is then redistributed to vital cells through a filter system that allows only one water molecule to be forcefully injected through a cluster of perforations that are wide enough to let in water, but nothing else. As the body becomes more and more dehydrated, the injection pressure gradually but forcefully rises. This rise in pressure is called hypertension.

The brain is dependent on this process of water delivery into its cells—at normal blood pressure readings. When alcohol shuts down this process, the brain cells get dehydrated and begin to signal their thirst by producing hangover headaches. Drinking one or two glasses of water before taking alcohol will prevent the post-alcohol headaches.

Alcohol is a diuretic. It forces water out of the body. It induces thirst. More of the same has to be taken when water is not the preferred choice for quenching thirst. Alcohol, by producing dehydration, will cause stress. Prolonged stress will cause production and release of the body's own morphine-like substances—endorphins and enkephalins. These "opiates of the body" are designed to prevent fear and anxiety from causing a sudden disruption of an activity, such as fighting or running away from danger. These elements give the body stamina to stay the course. Long-distance runners depend on the timely release of these compounds to finish a race. Increased production and release of the opiates becomes an addictive process. Long-distance runners get their high by running more, and alcoholics by drinking more of the same, establishing a conditioned reflex to increase the rate of endorphin release in the body.

Women, because they go through the monthly stress of menstruation, and from time to time the even greater physiological stress of pregnancy and childbirth, have more easily stimulated endorphin-manufacturing and -secreting mechanisms. When alcohol begins to enhance these mechanisms, addictive highs are achieved more readily than in men, whose bodies do not have the same readiness for production of their natural opiates. This is the simple reason why alcoholism can become established in women in one to three years from their first experience of mood manipulation with alcohol. In men, it may take several years before they become compulsive drinkers.

The great news for alcoholics, and even the users of hard drugs, is that water also stimulates the centers that register endorphins' effects. Water has a more direct effect as a stimulant than alcohol. Within minutes of drinking a glass of water, it stimulates the sympathetic nervous system and the serotonergic centers of the spinal column and the brain; they remain stimulated for up to two hours.

These are the nerve centers of the body that increase stamina and raise the pain threshold—what alcoholics and drug addicts try to achieve through substance abuse. This is the reason water is a natural pain medication. It is infinitely more effective as a painkiller than anything in the arsenal of the pharmaceutical industry, and it has no side effects. It surely does not kill you with its side effects, while taking pain medications is a gamble: Their side effects may kill without warning. Every year, about 8,000 people bleed to death from one traditional painkiller alone. The others cause liver damage and can easily cause death.

Water should be a medication of choice for people with pain. Water should become a medication of choice in those who wish to kick the addictive habits of alcohol intake or drug abuse. It will greatly increase your odds of success, if you are determined to kick the habit and regain the lost respect of family and friends. Here is one success story.

D. R. L. was a young lady of 35 when she wrote the following letter in 1997. She has a son. She became an alcoholic when she was in her 20s. Here is her story.

Dear Dr. Batmanghelidj:

My father introduced me to your water discoveries at a very critical time for me, and my infant son. I am 35 years old and had been alcoholic since my twenties. As with most people so afflicted, my personal relationships were rocky and impermanent, and I had a broken marriage behind me. I had also just reached the end of a follow-on relationship, in a fashion that was both shocking and stressful, since I was without resources to continue my life in a city strange to me. I got into Alcoholics Anonymous determined to prevent any repetitions of my agonies.

At this point, my father gave me your book and urged me to act on its content with full resolve. I did so, grasping at what I saw as an unexpected deliverance—like the hand of God. I was gratified to discover the power of water to still the cravings of an alcoholic. Soon I realized that alcoholism was really a thirst signal that I was habituated to respond to with alcohol, which is a powerful dehydrating agent. One became like a dog chasing its own tail. Dehydration through alcohol is self-perpetuating, unless the thirst sensations are answered with water.

Persevering with adequate daily water intake, and the elimination of dehydrating caffeinated drinks, I found myself able to deal effectively with my personal locational crisis. I was able to get my belongings and furniture together, rent a truck and load it, and drive myself and my son back to California from Las Vegas. My former, alcoholic self could not have done this. I resettled myself in California, went back successfully into my work as a beautician, and buckled down to raising my son.

Of course I still have normal problems like everyone else, but alcohol is not one of them. Water has lifted this curse from my life. As I write, I have been ten months "dry," and I have been able to reorganize my life rationally. Adequate daily water intake is the bedrock on which to rebuild a life deranged by alcohol, and to help others to do the same. There are other benefits that will have great appeal to all alcoholic women, in particular.

As an alcoholic, I had begun to lose my youthful looks. Steady self-poisoning and dehydration with alcohol dulled and aged my complexion. In recent years, my weight had steadily increased for the reasons outlined so clearly in your book. I began to look puffy and pallid. Therefore I was elated— absolutely "stoked"—when rehydration caused my excess weight to just disappear. I could not believe it, and neither could my friends, as I regained the perfect figure I had enjoyed as a young woman. I did not have to "sweat" this, it just happened. My complexion began to change back to a wonderful, youthful glow that everyone remarks on, and which has delighted my father. My regained radiance is a big asset in my professional work as a beautician. The weight loss and adequate daily water intake invigorated my whole being. I began running on what you call "hydro-electric power," in your book.

With these changes came an overall renewal of life and outlook. I continued to help others through AA. I began attracting life-positive gentlemen of purpose and substance, instead of the lesser fellows who would tolerate an alcoholic woman. Church attendance brought me comfort, and I wanted to attend. I plan and work for an ever-improving life. Reviewing my past from my normalized perspective, I apologized to my father for my many years of outrages, and for the suffering I had caused him because of his love for me. Dad had almost given up on me, but his provision of your book was decisive in my redemption.

My father tells everyone that you are one of the greatest physicians in the history of the world. I think he is right. Thank you Dr. Batmanghelidj, for all you have done, not alone for me with my turnaround of life, but for all mankind.

Very sincerely yours, D. R. L.

The information on water empowered D. R. L. to kick a habit that would normally be much stronger than you read in this uplifting letter. This book is designed to empower you to prevent dehydration, and thereby prevent the various diseases that are produced by persistent unintentional dehydration, with particular focus on the deadliest diseases of dehydration: obesity, depression, and cancer.

You now know that water can replace the urge to drink alcohol: Alcohol cannot be a substitute for the water needs of the body.

CAFFEINATED BEVERAGES

In my opinion, this is the most important chapter in this book. My hope is that the information I am sharing will establish a new mind-set in you. This is why I am giving so much detailed explanation rather than writing a few paragraphs of general information. My aim is to shed a new light on the fluids you may be drinking—fluids your body is not able to handle without getting hurt. After you read this chapter, the choice is yours to make: Pursue a prudent approach to better health, or follow the lifestyle of the vast majority in our society, who are unwittingly poisoning themselves with the wrong beverages.

The tea shrub was discovered in China thousands of years ago and is now being grown in many parts of the world. The active ingredient in tea is caffeine; its color comes from tannic acid. Tannic acid is used to harden and cure leather.

The coffee bean was discovered on the Arabian subcontinent. Shepherds in the region realized its stimulating effect on their goats. Goats climb trees and eat anything they can chew, even paper. They harm growing plants by eating even their roots. Legend has it that goats that ate the coffee bean would not sleep at night and would be agitated and frisky. The local shepherds reported their discovery of the effects of coffee berries to the local priors. One of these wanted to use the berries to see if he could keep awake and pray without falling asleep. Thus, coffee was introduced to the world.

Guru nuts (Cola acuminata), from which cola drinks are made, had been a favorite "chew" in Sudan for many centuries. The cola drinks we use in America get their taste from guru nuts. The active ingredient in this nut is caffeine. When using this nut to make cola, more caffeine is added to the recipe to standardize the stimulant effect of the beverages.

In 1850 only 1.6 8-ounce containers of soda were consumed per person per year in the United States. In late 1980s more than 500 12-ounce cans of sodas were consumed per person per year. The 1994 annual report of the beverage industry showed that per capita consumption of sodas was 49.1 gallons per year. Of this, 28.2 percent was diet sodas. Eighty-four percent of all sodas consumed belonged to two companies, Coca-Cola (48.2 percent) and Pepsi-Cola (35.9 percent). Of this 84 percent share of the market, only 5.5 percent are caffeine-free diet sodas. A vast number of people are drinking caffeinated sodas.

The beverage industry thrives on the addictive properties of caffeine. A report published in The Nation, April 27, 1998, states: "The most conservative estimates have children and teens guzzling more than sixty-four gallons of soda a year—an amount that has tripled for teens since 1978, doubled for the 6–11 set and increased by a quarter for under-5 tots (from a 1994 survey by the Agriculture Department)." The Washington Post of Sunday, May 30, 2004, reveals that obesity has doubled in adults and kids between 8 and 11 years of age and has tripled in adolescents. This finding confirms what I published several years ago in my book *Your Body's Many Cries for Water*. It is also interesting to note that the increased consumption of sodas by children younger than five years probably explains why the rate of asthma occurrence in that age group tripled between 1980 and 1994.

The beverage industry's recent introduction of new brands—Surge, Zapped, Full Speed, Outburst, Josta, all laced with caffeine and the pick-me-up herb guarana, which hypes "raw primal power"—is designed to entice children and teenagers to consume more and more sodas. The 12-ounce cans of soda that contain high amounts of caffeine include Jolt (72 mg), XTC (70 mg), Pepsi-Cola's Josta (58 mg), and Coca-Cola's Surge (51 mg). And you get a near double dose when you buy the 20-ounce bottles.

At school, kids often drink sodas in place of milk, and the schools profit from the sale of these addictive beverages. They serve the regular 12-ounce cans of soda, with Mountain Dew containing 55 mg of caffeine per can, Coke containing 45 mg, Sunkist 40 mg, and Pepsi 37 mg. Grown-ups consume so much coffee that coffee bars are sprouting like mushrooms. It is said that a 12-ounce cup of regular Starbucks coffee contains 190 mg of caffeine.

It is my professional opinion that caffeine by itself has all the detrimental effects on the brain cells to produce the type of brain physiology that dislocates the brain from stimuli received from the outside. In addition, the dehydration caused by extensive caffeine intake produces numerous health problems—among them asthma and allergies—devastatingly early. Thus, my protocol for the treatment of asthma excludes any form of caffeine-containing beverage until the body has recovered from caffeine's unhealthy side effects, particularly on the brain and nervous system. After that, wisdom will have to take over.

A survey at Pennsylvania State University showed that some students drank 14 cans of soda a day. One girl had consumed 37 Cokes in two days. Many admitted they could not live without these soft drinks. If deprived, these people would develop withdrawal symptoms, very much like those of people addicted to other drugs. Boys Life magazine surveyed its readers and found that 8 percent drink eight or more sodas a day. The administrators of one Boy Scout jamboree collected 200,000 empty cans for recycling. A Soft Drink Association survey of the use of soft drinks in hospitals in America found that 85 percent serve sodas with patients' meals.

The increase of soda consumption by children under five is a significant event. In my opinion this has a direct relationship to increased occurrence of obesity and asthma in children. Occurrence of asthma in children tripled between 1980 and 1994, and obesity in children has now become a national crisis—another impact of excessive soda consumption in this sector of society.

CAFFEINE IS A DRUG

Caffeine, one of the main components of most sodas, is a drug. It has addictive properties because of its direct action on the brain. It also acts on the kidneys and causes increased urine production. Caffeine has diuretic properties. It is physiologically a dehydrating agent. This is the main reason why a person can drink many cans of soda every day and never be satisfied. The water does not stay in the body long enough. At the same time, many people confuse their feelings of thirst with hunger: Thinking they have consumed enough "water" in the soda, they begin to eat more food than their body needs, when in fact the body's only need is for natural water. Thus the dehydration caused by caffeine-containing sodas can over time lead to gradual weight gain.

Caffeine has "pick-me-up" properties. It stimulates the brain and body even when you're exhausted! It seems that caffeine disrupts the strict control mechanism governing the use of energy from its stockpiles in the cells, particularly the brain cells. Under the influence of caffeine, the reserve of energy stored in the cells for emergency purposes is used up for trivial functions. The functions that would not normally gain access to these energy reserves, when the stockpiles are low, do so under caffeine's influence. You might think this is a good thing. It may be for emergency needs, but drawing from the energy reserves of vital cells in the body day in and day out is the root of many health problems in our caffeine-consuming society.

CAFFEINE IS A PLANT POISON

The plants that make caffeine, and even morphine and cocaine, have refined their manufacturing processes for a particular purpose: to create nerve poisons for use against their predators. Why do you think people who use cocaine and morphine get hooked and often die? It's due to the impact of these chemicals on users' nervous systems.

Through eons of time, plants developed these poisons as a way to eliminate any grazing animal that would feast on their foliage. It is a matter of life and death for the plant. Without such defenses, the plants would become extinct in no time.

Field animals have learned to give these plants a bye. Grazing sheep skirt the colorful poppy in favor of less harmful foliage. It is interesting that some animal species have used the same poison-making technique for their own survival. Frogs are delectable food for reptiles. However, some species of frog manufacture very potent poisons in their bodies. These poisons are deposited in their skin in the form of exotically colored patches of pigmentation. This is how frogs survive next to a very high population of reptiles per square mile in the Amazon rain forest. The art of poison making in nature is highly refined. Even mushrooms are good at it.

Caffeine in the leaves of the tea plant and beans of coffee plant is in the same category: It's a poison that plants manufacture to protect their presence on this planet. Caffeine works through the nervous system of whatever ingests it by inhibiting the action of an enzyme called phospho-diesterase (phospho di-ester-aze) in the nerve cells.

Activation of this enzyme is a pivotal step in the process of memory formation and its retention. The inhibition of this enzyme in the critters that would eat caffeine is intended to produce euphoria; rob them of their established knowledge of dangers they might confront; induce forgetfulness to use their art of camouflage; diminish their alertness and quick reaction to relocate to a more protected area. In this way, the caffeine-producing plants would deliver to their consumers the kiss of death, by making them vulnerable and easily caught and eaten by their own natural food-chain predators.

The existence of food-chain predators is not exclusive to insects; it includes the higher animals too. In humans, competing for survival in the rat race of society is no less a task than survival among more primitive forms of life.

For example, it is now realized that children who drink caffeine-containing sodas in place of water achieve a much lower grade average in the school than children who only drink water. One-group gets Cs and Fs and the other group gets As. and Bs. This is now a known fact. Without realizing the origin of the problem, the impact of drinking soda in place of water has given rise to attention deficit hyperactivity disorder (ADHD). The suffering of this disorder's young victims is another outcome of caffeine consumption in our society. Do these children have the same chance of survival and success in their future as those who do not consume caffeine? Definitely not! These children will be given strong drugs and become a constant source of concern for their parents and teachers in their shortened lives.

Although most books on drugs point to the immediate effects of caffeine on the brain, none of them discusses its long-term impact on the physiology of the brain, which must adjust for the dehydration and the phospho-diesterase suppression caffeine causes.

DIET SODAS CAN CAUSE WEIGHT GAIN

My observation has been that diet sodas, even though they contain no appreciable number of calories, are possibly the cause of weight gain in people who resort to taking them to control their weight. This paradox needs explanation. The following is the result of my research into this enigma.

Most of us assume that manufactured beverages can replace water in the body. Because these beverages contain water, we believe our bodies will be adequately served. This assumption is wrong. The recent broad-based increase in consumption of mainly caffeine-containing sodas is background to many of our current health problems.

The confusion that all manufactured beverages will supply the body with its daily water needs, more than any other cause, is responsible for some of the diseases that we encounter. Gross dis-figurement of the body by fat collection is the initial step in the decline of the human body, and in my opinion is caused by the wrong choice of fluids intake. Some beverages do more damage than others. When sodas contain sugar, at least some of the brain's need for sugar is satisfied. If caffeine is releasing ATP (adenosine triphosphate) energy to enhance performance, at least its sugar companion will replenish some of the lost ATP, even if the final result is a deficit expenditure of ATP by the brain.

In the early 1980s, however, a new product was introduced into the beverage industry—aspartame. Aspartame is 180 times as sweet as sugar without any calories. It is now in common use because the FDA has deemed it safe to use in place of sugar. In a very short peri-od of time it has been incorporated in more than 5,000 products.

In the intestinal tract, aspartame converts to two highly excita-tory neurotransmitter amino acids, aspartate and phenylalanine, as well as methyl alcohol/formaldehyde—wood alcohol. About 10 percent of the aspartame consumed in foods becomes formaldehyde and methyl alcohol. It is claimed that the liver ren-ders methyl alcohol nontoxic. I think this claim brushes aside serious concerns about a manufactured "food" that has a known toxic by-product.

Formaldehyde and methyl alcohol have been cited in medical pub-lications as producing eye-nerve damage, to the point of blindness. The recent rise in macular degeneration and retinopathy, even in the comparatively younger sector of our population, is being blamed on the excessive use of artificial sweeteners.

Other secondary complications of the use of the sweetener aspar-tame are tumor formation in the brain and secondary neurological disorders. Dr. H. J. Roberts of West Palm Beach, Florida, has done much research on the adverse effects of aspartame. He has identi-fied a number of "aspartame diseases." In his June 2002 article pub-lished in Townsend Letter for Doctors and Patients, Dr. Roberts listed a number of neurological problems that have been produced by aspartame. He has a collection of 1,200 patients who developed neurological complication through the use of aspartame: 43 percent had headaches; 31 percent had dizziness and unsteadiness; 31 percent had confusion and memory loss; 13 percent had drowsiness and sleepiness; 11 percent had major epileptic convulsions; 3 percent had minor epileptic attacks and "absences of the mind"; 10 percent had severe slurring of speech; 8 percent had severe tremors; 6 percent had severe "hyperactivity" and "restless legs"; 6 percent had atypical facial pains. He reports that after cutting out aspartame, these people improved. As you might know, methyl alcohol and formaldehyde damage to the brain cells and the optic nerve is unfortunately irreversible.

It goes without saying that the FDA has exposed society to a host of health problems by permitting the use of aspartame. Some people could be exposed to detrimental levels of formaldehyde and methyl alcohol as a result of drinking a few diet sodas daily. Unfortunately, the neurotoxic effects of formaldehyde and methyl alcohol in the body are cumulative.

Like caffeine, aspartame attacks the energy stockpile of the brain. The spent fuel residues (GMP and AMP) trigger hunger mechanisms. It is a well-recognized scientific fact that spent fuel AMP does cause hunger. Thus: "diet sodas cause indiscriminate overuse of energy reserves of cells in the brain and produce more spent fuel dumps that would trigger further overeating."

Caffeine causes addiction, and people who consume it on a regular basis should be assumed to be addicts. Hence, caffeinated diet sodas in sedentary people must cause weight gain; they indirectly stimulate more food intake because of the brain's forced use of its energy reserves. Bear in mind, only 20 percent of the energy contained in the foods we eat will reach the brain. The rest will be stored in the form of fat, if not used by muscle activity. This weight gain is one of many effects of diet soda consumption.

More important is the brain's naturally established reaction to sweet taste. The jargon used is *cephalic phase response*. A conditioned reflex gets established as a result of lifelong experience with sweet taste. When sweet taste stimulates the tongue, the brain programs the liver to prepare for acceptance of new energy—sugar—from outside. The liver in turn stops the manufacture of sugar from the protein and starch reserves of the body and instead begins to store the metabolic fuels that are circulating in the blood. Michael Tardoff, Mark Friedman, and other scientists have shown that cephalic phase response alters the metabolic activity in favor of nutrient storage; the fuel available for conversion is reduced, and this leads to the development of appetite.

If it is indeed sugar that stimulates the response, the effect on the liver will be to regulate what has entered the body. However, if sweet taste is not followed by nutrient availability, an urge to eat will be the outcome. The liver produces the signals and the urge to eat. The more a sweet taste without the accompanying calories stimulates the taste buds, the more there is an urge to eat.

The relationship of cephalic phase response to sweet taste has been clearly shown in animal models through the use of saccharin. Using aspartame, several scientists have shown a similar urge to overeat in humans. Blundel and Hill have shown that non-nutritive sweeteners—aspartame in solution—will enhance appetite and increase short-term food intake. They report, "after ingestion of aspartame, the volunteers were left with a residual hunger compared with what they reported after glucose. This residual hunger is functional; it leads to increased food consumption."

Tardoff and Friedman have shown that this urge to eat more food after artificial sweeteners can last up to 90 minutes after the sweet drink, even when all blood tests show normal values. Even when blood levels for insulin—which is thought to be the cause of hunger—achieved normal range, the test animals consume more food than the control batch. What this means is that the brain retains for a long time the urge to eat when the taste buds for sugar are stimulated without sugar having entered the system. The sweet taste will cause the brain to program the liver to store supplies rather than release supplies from its storage.

Basically, people who consume diet sodas to reduce weight may suffer from the paradoxical response of their body to repeated stimulation of the taste buds with sugar substitutes by getting fatter than before.

I know of many diet soda drinkers who began to gain weight. One stands out, a young man in his 20s, about 5 feet, 5 inches tall. He used to drink soda regularly—just like many college students, under constant pressure to complete their work. He had already gained excess weight by the time he graduated. After graduation, to reduce weight, he began drinking diet sodas, eight cans per day. In about two years he must have gained another 30 pounds. He seemed to be as round as he was tall. Walking became difficult; he seemed to have to swing his hip to take a step. He also drank his diet soda at meals and ate more than his body needed.

I am happy to report that this young man stopped consuming sodas three years ago and has become trim and healthy. Of course, he has also begun exercising very seriously.

Aspartate and Phenylalanine

When caffeine and aspartame are introduced into the body, they stimulate the cell physiology in the brain, the liver, the kidneys, the pancreas, the endocrine glands, and so on. Aspartame is converted to the amino acids phenylalanine and aspartate. Both have direct stimulatory effects on the brain. The sum total of the effect of caffeine and aspartame very quickly establishes a new mode of activity for the brain, because these neuroactive amino acids are available frequently and in larger quantities than the other naturally available amino acids that would otherwise establish a balanced physiology.

Most neurotransmitters are secondary products from one or another amino acid. However, aspartate is one of a pair of unique amino acids that don't need to be converted to a secondary product to act on the brain. There are receiving points (receptors) for these two amino acids—aspartate and glutamate—on certain nerve cells that influence body physiology very dramatically.

The use of artificial sweeteners for their false stimulation of nerve terminals that register the entry of energy supplies into the body has more severe repercussions than simply causing an increase in weight. These chemicals constantly swing the body physiology in the direction dictated by the nerve system. Using them without a thorough understanding of their long-term effects in the body is shortsighted. My understanding of the micro physiology within cells leaves me concerned about the long-term effect of the stimulation of the nerve/glandular systems in the brain through artificial sweeteners.

Research has shown that receptors for aspartate are abundantly present on some nerve systems whose products also stimulate the reproductive organs and the breasts. A constant stimulation of the breast glands without the other factors associated with pregnancy may well be implicated in the rise in the rate of breast cancer in women. I have no doubt that the aspartame-induced excess prolactin production plays a major role in the increased frequency of breast cancers in women. One of the less explored complications of aspartame may be its effect as a possible facilitator in brain cancer formation. Fed to rats, aspartame has been implicated in brain tumor formation.

As has been explained so far, the human body has many different indicators when it runs short of water. At these times, it needs only water. It will complicate matters if you give your body artificially taste-enhanced fluids on a regular basis.

Caffeine is similarly an addictive drug, the use of which is legal.

Children in particular become vulnerable to the addictive properties of caffeine-containing beverages. Stimulating the body with pleasure-enhancing chemicals at the early stages of a child's life may program the senses to the use of drugs—perhaps harder addictive drugs when the child reaches school age.

You now have an idea of the difference between water and other beverages as far as better health is concerned. You are aware that beverages on the market may have serious detrimental effects on the health and wellness of those who buy into the advertising hype of their manufacturers. In the pages to come, I will explain how water shortage in the body can translate to excess fat, to the point of disease.

CHAPTER 3

THE LIFE-GIVING PROPERTIES OF WATER

If eating is about providing energy for the human body, water is more important as a source of energy than anything else we eat. This is where confusion has arisen in the application of science to human behavior. All our health problems stem from the misconception that food is the only source of energy to the human body. We speak of the hydrolysis of this or that element in the body— the term refers to the breakdown of a substance through the action of water—yet we have never realized that the chemical processes involve the transfer of energy from water to whatever that is being broken down.

Scientists George and associates have studied the formula for energy transfer from water, and have shown that hydrolysis adds one zero—increases by one order of magnitude—to the energy content of a substance in the process of breaking it down. It's a bit like dripping oil on top of a piece of wood that has a hard time burning: You stimulate the burning process and get a more intense fire. In the body, chemical reactions become more intense when water is available. George et al. have shown that the energy content in a standard weight of magnesium-ATP, which is 600 Joule units before it is broken down, becomes 5,850 Joule units when it is hydrolyzed. Thus, as I see it, the chemical reactions that take place in our bodies constantly because of the action of water energize the body by one order of magnitude.

The formula for this chemical reaction, and its energy calculation by George and associates, is shown below.

IN LIVING CELLS

WATER

IS THE PRIMARY SOURCE OF ENERGY

$$MgATP^{2-} + H_2O = ADP^{3-}/ADPH^{2-} + Mg^{2+}/H^+ + H_2PO_4^-/HPO_4^{2-}$$

$$600 \qquad 1500 \quad 600 \quad 998 \quad 1168 \quad 318 \quad 1251$$

The units of energy are measured in Kilo Joules

(Energy required to raise the temperature of
one pound of water through 1 F*= 1 J)

Taking this newly understood effect of hydrolysis to its logical conclusion, a total reevaluation of our understanding of the human metabolism becomes unavoidable. For example, if one egg possesses about 70 calories, when the body begins to hydrolyze and metabolize the components of the egg, the output of energy from its metabolism may reach about 700 calories. Not having taken into consideration the energizing effect of water in the chemical reactions of the body, the traditional evaluation of the energy consumption of the body for its myriad chemical reactions suffers from inaccuracy and underestimation. This is why we have failed to consider the need to hydrate the body before any food intake—hence the many unsolved health problems in modern medical science.

Now you know water is the primary source of energy in all chemical reactions associated with food metabolism of the body. You now understand the wisdom of making water available to prepare the body for receiving food and processing its components. Food is similar to fossil fuel in traditional power plants; it is "dirty" energy and has much residue. The outcome of relying more on food as the primary source of energy is disease: obesity, cholesterol deposits, diabetes, hypertension, depression, neurological disorders such as multiple sclerosis, Alzheimer's disease, Parkinson's disease, various cancers, and many, many more.

Hydroelectricity:
The Preferred Source of Energy
for All Body Functions

Water has yet another infinitely more important role in energy formation in the body. It is responsible for the manufacture of hydroelectricity, primarily for the functions of the brain. This form of energy is "clean"—it has almost no residue or waste products. Excess water is excreted in form of urine. It does not stay in the body in form of a "lake," the way excess food forms mountains of fat. The hydroelectric form of energy is much more suited to the delicate metabolism of the brain.

It is uncanny the way water is used to make electricity inside the cells to energize the intricate functions that keep the cells alive and productive. Certain proteins are found within the membranes of every cell in the body. These proteins have an affinity for certain minerals available in the blood circulation and the solution surrounding the cells. Some of these proteins collect sodium and potassium, some magnesium, and some calcium. These minerals, when attached to their specific protein, get spun by the rush of water and begin to shift with the fast rotation of the protein.

This process manufactures electricity that gets stored in the membrane stockpiles known as ATP or GTP (guanosine triphosphate). In this energy-generating process, the appropriate minerals are also relocated to balance the osmotic ratio between the outside and inside of the cells. Philippa M. Wiggin has described the funda-

> Philippa M, Wiggin has shown that the mechanism that controls or brings about the effective function of the cation pumps utilizes the energy transforming property of water, the solvent; "The source of energy for cation transport or ATP synthesis lies in increases in chemical potentials with increasing hydration of small cations and polyphosphate

anions in the highly structured interfacial aqueous phase of the two phosphorylated intermediates[1]". Waiting to get thirsty, when the body fluids become concentrated before thirst is induced, one loses the energy-generating properties of water in the dehydrated cells of the body. This is a major reason why we should prevent dehydration, rather than wait to correct it. This new understanding of the role of water in cation exchange is enough justification to let the body engage in prudent surplus water management rather than forcing it into drought and deficit water management. 1- Wiggins PM; A Mechanism of ATP-Driven Cation Pumps; PP-266-269, Biophysics of Water, Eds. Felix Franks and Sheila F. Mathis, John Wiley and Sons, Ltd. 1982

mentals of this process.

The fact that it is the interior of the body's cells that becomes drastically dehydrated when the body is short of water is the most important phenomenon to understand. In dehydration, 66 percent of the water loss is from the interior of the cells, 26 percent of the loss is from extracellular fluid volume, and only 8 percent is borne by the blood tissue in the vascular system, which constricts within its network of capillaries and maintains the integrity of the circulation system. Thus, dehydrated cells begin to run low on energy reserves and begin to suffer. They begin to reflect their dehydration by producing various symptoms of inefficient performance in the routine functions of the body. The brain is the most vulnerable organ of the body to this problem.

There are about nine trillion brain and nerve cells in the body. They constantly communicate with one another to keep the body in sync with its environment. As it happens, the best and preferred source of clean energy they use for these complicated activities is hydroelectric energy. This is the reason a glass of water is the best pick-me-up drink you could imagine. It will energize the brain out of its listlessness in a matter of minutes. If you were to tap into the energy of food for this purpose, not only you would need water to digest the food for its eventual use, but the process would also take quite a long time: First the food is converted to sugar, and then the sugar is used by the brain cells as a source of energy.

The human brain is roughly 1/50 of the total body weight, and as I mentioned, it is said to possess about nine trillion nerve cells (computer chips). The brain cells are said to be 85 percent water. Twenty percent of blood circulation is allocated and made available to the brain. This means that the brain gets to pick and choose from the circulating blood what is needed for its normal functions. The brain puts the body to sleep, but does not shut itself off at night. It works all the time, just like the heart, the lungs, the liver, the glands, the blood circulation, and so on. It processes all the information from different parts of the body, as well as whatever enters it from daily exposure to its physical, social, and electromagnetic environment.

To process all these inputs and alert all parts of the body for a coordinated response, the brain expends a vast quantity of energy. At the same time, it expends energy in manufacturing the primary chemical messengers (neurotransmitters), which must then be transported to nerve endings. The transportation system uses a vast quantity of energy. This high rate of energy consumption by the brain is, in my opinion, the main reason it receives about 20 percent of blood circulation: It needs the water that the blood tissue contains to make hydroelectricity. Naturally, water will also bring the pick of the raw materials the brain needs to manufacture its chemicals.

There is a threshold for energy release for some inputs. The brain calculates and understands what is important and what is not for its energy expenditure. When ATP reserves are low, many stimuli do not invoke a response. This low ATP reserve in some overactive brain cells will become reflected as a fatigue state in the functions that are controlled by those brain cells. This is why food is not a good immediate pick-me-up, but water is.

The central control system in the brain happens to recognize the

low energy levels available for its functions. The sensations of
thirst or hunger also stem from low ready-to-access energy levels.
To mobilize energy from what's stored in the fat, hormonal release
mechanisms are needed. This takes a while longer (and requires
some physical activity for energy release) than the urgent needs of
the brain. The front of the brain gets energy either from hydroelectricity or from sugar in blood circulation.

THE BRAIN'S NEED FOR WATER
IS CONSTANT AND URGENT:

- One, to form hydroelectric energy for message transmission.

- Two, because the transport systems across the cell membranes
  of the brain depend on adequate water. The membrane barriers need to be more "fluid" so that transport of materials from
  blood to brain could take place more easily.

- Three, because the energy from hydroelectricity is also
  needed for all transport systems in the "water channels"
  within the nerves that connect the brain to different parts
  of the body.

These are three main reasons why the brain tissue is 85 percent
water, and is almost always thirsty. If you confuse this brain thirst
for hunger just because the sensations are similar, you will create a
physiological state conducive to premature aging, disease, decay,
and early death. Obesity, depression, and cancer are three of the
labels we in medicine have created to describe the killer process of
persistent unintentional dehydration in the human body.

In a dehydrated state, the human body begins to initially inhibit
some functions and eventually dismantle its structures and components. As an example, consider the two forms of diabetes. In type
II diabetes, insulin production and release is inhibited. In type I
diabetes the insulin-producing beta-cells are destroyed from inside.
Both forms of diabetes are the direct consequence of unintentional dehydration—better still, medical ignorance about the impor-

tance of water to health and well-being. The body has no alternative but to deal strictly and economically with problems of dehydration. Thus, there is a metabolic component to dehydration that we must understand in order to reverse a disease process. When I use the word dehydration, I'm not referring to water shortage only; I'm also speaking of the shortage of raw materials that culminates in a disease state. This will be explained in the sections on depression and cancer.

CHAPTER 4

HOW DOES DEHYDRATION
CAUSE EXCESS WEIGHT?

YOU OVEREAT WHEN YOU ARE THIRSTY!

The sensations of thirst and hunger are generated simultaneously to indicate the brain's needs for energy supply. We do not recognize the sensation of thirst and interpret both indicators as the urge to eat. We eat food even when the body should receive water, the infinitely cleaner source of energy.

Storage of energy in the energy pools in the brain, and in the absence of adequate generation of hydroelectricity seems to rely heavily on the availability of sugar. The brain has to constantly collect sugar from the blood to replenish its ATP and GTP stockpiles.

To satisfy the brain's immediate energy requirements, the human body has developed a very delicate balancing system to keep a normal range of sugar concentration in the blood. It does this in two ways: first, by stimulating the intake of proteins and starch that are easily converted into sugar, as well as any form of sugar that might also be taken in the diet; and second, by converting some starch and proteins from the stored reserves of the body into sugar. This latter mechanism of converting protein to sugar is called gluco-neo-genesis. It means remaking of sugar from other materials. This remanufacturing of sugar for use by the brain is done in the liver. When this process is still inadequate, the body begins reluctantly to dive into its fat stores and convert or even metabolize fat itself for energy production.

In our society, we have developed a sweet tooth for immediate satis-
faction of the brain. Many cultures, such as the Chinese, have avoided this cultural pitfall. In the West, however, we consume a lot of sugary foods. In such situation, when the body receives a good supply of
"sweetness," the liver begins to initially store the extra sugar in form of
starch, and subsequently in form of fat. Glycogen is made of a very
long-chain of glucose molecules that are connected together in the
form of a "polymer." It is stored in the liver and the muscle tissue.
Glycogen is the readily usable starch that can very quickly be converted—one or two glucose molecules at a time—into ATP when the
ATP reserves of the cells in the body are beginning to get depleted.

Since only 20 percent of the circulation reaches the brain, only 20
percent of the sugar in circulation is used up; the remaining 80 percent is stored in the liver and fat cells. Beyond what the liver stores
as glycogen, excess sugar is converted into fat and released into the
blood circulation to be stored by the fat cells. Fat cells also collect
sugar and convert it to fat independently of the liver. This is why I
call food taken for brain energy "dirty fuel." In normal circumstances, food should be balanced for the repair of wear and tear and
the manufacturing needs of the body, and not as the primary and
only source of brain energy—the brain exercises priority for its
needed supplies over the rest of the organs in the body. Water
should be available to manufacture "local" hydroelectricity for the
constantly active brain cells.

When there is not enough sugar in circulation, the liver begins to
manufacture it and constantly tops up the blood levels by the addition of more sugar. In the beginning, it will convert stored starch,
followed by proteins and small quantities of fat. Initially, fat conversion is a very slow process.

The body needs to go without starchy food for some time before a
higher rate of fat breakdown and its metabolism is established.
Starchy foods and high sugar content of the diet inhibit the
enzyme systems that initiate the breakdown of fat in the fat stores.

Proteins are more accessible and broken down more easily than fat. The main proteins in circulation that will be used up are albumin, globulin, and fibrinogen. The rate of their manufacture by the liver, and their breakdown, will initially tip the balance in the direction of more breakdown than manufacture.

The next source of protein for conversion into sugar is loose proteins held in reserve in the liver and other cells of the body. The muscle mass itself is the last source of energy to be attacked.

By the time the muscle mass has to be broken down, fat-burning enzymes will have come to the rescue. Nonetheless, some muscle tissue is lost in severe dehydration, and uninformed dieting.

Fat deposits are made up of many single units of fatty acids joined together. It is the individual fatty acids that are broken for their energy value. Each gram of fat gives 9 calories of energy. Each gram of protein or sugar provides only 4 calories of energy. This is why, when fat is metabolized, you feel far less hungry.

There is a major problem with breaking down the muscle tissue on and off, as occurs in yo-yo dieting. Each time muscle is broken down into its chemical component for conversion to energy, much of the minerals stored in the muscle tissue will be lost. Two of the most vital items that get shed are vitamin B6 and zinc, the depletion of which will have very serious effects. For those of you who need to know how: Each molecule of myoglobin that holds on to iron for its oxygen-binding qualities is composed of four pyrrole rings, which cradle one molecule of iron among them. When this composition is dismantled in muscle tissue breakdown, each pyrrole ring will attach to one molecule of B6 and one zinc atom, and drag them out of the body—other very precious minerals such as selenium, magnesium, manganese, and more, are also lost.

Replacement of zinc and B6 lost from the body reserves is not as easy as their loss. When you lose 1 pound of muscle mass, and you are happy with the lower reading on the scale, you have lost much from your body's mineral reserves. When you do this frequently with yo-yo dieting, losing a few pounds of weight at a time, you do much harm to your own body.

You need adequate zinc supply for rejuvenation of your body cells, when mature cells create daughter cells and then die. Thus, shortage of zinc in the body reserves will prevent rejuvenation and cause premature aging. As for B6, this particular vitamin is absolutely vital for normal brain function. It is essential for conversion of some amino acids to their respective neurotransmitters. The health problems that emerge as a result of the B6 and zinc depletion in the body include depression—and most other emotional problems—as well as the major chronic pains, diabetes, hypertension, and imbalance in the function of the endocrine glands, to name a few. I will discuss this subject more fully in the chapter on using water as a preventive medication.

BROWN FAT AS OPPOSED TO WHITE FAT

In children, fat stores are brown in color and have much blood circulation in them. In this brown fat, fat is metabolized directly and heat is generated. This is the reason children can withstand cold weather much more comfortably than older people. In the later years of life, fat stores have less blood circulation; they become white and are less accessible to the enzymes that would mobilize the fatty acids for use in the liver and the muscles. Nonetheless, even fat deposits in the fat stores are recycled in two to three weeks. It is not as if once fat is collected and stored, the body forgets it is there. The body continuously refreshes these stores. The old fats are broken down, and new fats are made to replace the old fat "lumps." It is within this process that we could change the recycling process in favor of less formation and more breakdown of fat from the fat stores of the body.

Within the natural design and development of each animal species, and because of its lower-weight/higher-energy ratio and tremendous protective and insulating properties against trauma and cold, storing fat for its energy value became established as a multipurpose survival strategy. Fat cells are designed to pick up the excess of energy-laden carbohydrate and lipid products and store them within their interior in the form of fat aggregates or "lumps of fat." This process has two major advantages. First, the blood level of certain elements will remain within a healthier norm— such as keeping the amount of sugar in blood circulation at a non-toxic level. Second, the stored fat is then released only when the body is in definite need of it for energy. This stored fat is not released willy-nilly. There is a physiological rule to its conversion to the smaller particles of fat and their use as energy.

Fat is a high-energy product that is stored in different tissues to be used when the energy supply from outside the body becomes erratic or diminished. Fat is stored in specially designed fat cells that pick up the excess sugar in circulation and convert it to fatty acids, which are lumped together to form triglycerides—chunks of fat. To reuse this stored fat, it has to be broken back into individual fatty acids once again and released as free fatty acids in circulation, to be picked up by the tissues that are short of energy. Breakdown of fat depends on the presence of water. One unit of water has to be sacrificed to separate one unit of fatty acid from its connection to the "chain." The process is called hydrolysis of fat. Hydrolysis of fat is under the control of an enzyme called lipase. This is why we need to drink water regularly and often to supply its free form for the breakdown of fat. Water will also indirectly stimulate the lipase that breaks up fat.

To understand the fat-breakdown process in relationship to eating, you need to understand the following physiological events:

- Lipase gets activated when the level of sugar available to fat cells falls lower than is normally present in circulation.

- Peaking the blood sugar by the intake of sweet snacks or starchy foods, which immediately get converted to sugar and cause insulin release, will inhibit the lipase activity.

- Lipase activity is also brought about by the release of many hormones and neurotransmitters. This variety of lipase is known as hormone-sensitive lipase. Adrenalin and noradren-alin (norepinephrine) are by far the most potent of the lipase activators. Growth hormone, other adrenal gland hormones, and thyroid hormone are other potent activators of lipase.

- In the absence or very short supply of carbohydrates, and when the stored glycogen is getting used up, the body prefer-entially metabolizes fat from its stores for energy formation.

- Normally, 40 to 50 percent of the calories in a good diet are from fat. In any case, much of the carbohydrate eaten is con-verted into fatty acids and metabolized gradually throughout the day, unless the system is loaded with successive carbohy-drate intake. Often, this is the result of confusion between feeling thirsty and hungry, when you eat instead of quench-ing your thirst with water.

- The energy formed from one molecule of sugar is much less than the energy formed from one molecule of fat. One gram-molecule of sugar forms 38 units of ATP from 66 percent of energy in the sugar, and the other 34 percent is converted to heat; one molecule of fat forms 146 units. Thus, fat burning is more energy-efficient than burning carbohydrates. Think about it: The body knows how to store energy. What we want to do is learn how to tap into that energy without letting it accumulate excessively to the point of distorting the shape of the body. Water seems to be the ideal "solution" for this problem.

- The liver is fully capable of desaturating fatty acids for ready use in the architectural structure of membranes. The triglyc-eride content of the liver consists mainly of its unsaturated variety, whereas the rest of the fat stores of the body are formed from the saturated fatty acids. This information brings into question the validity of the conventional views on essen-tial fatty acids, even though in the past I have also subscribed to those views. Here you see the true value of an open mind in scientific research. I no longer worry about the kind of fat I eat. I enjoy my generous helpings of butter with the knowl-edge that my liver will take care of the rest.

- Fat is a most important element for human survival. In the water environment of the interior of the body, fat plays an indispensable and vital insulating role as fatty acids, cholesterol, and phospholipids. Both starch and proteins are water-soluble and will not be able to protect the architecture of the cells from getting out of shape and distorted.

- Eighty percent of cholesterol formed in the liver is eventually converted into bile salts, secreted into the biliary tract, and passed on into the intestine. The other 20 percent is converted into phospholipids and passed into the blood circulation.

- Cholesterol, apart from its use in the cell membrane of the brain and nerve tissues, is further converted into most of the sex hormones, secondary neurotransmitters (such as the array of prostaglandins, prostacyclins, and thromboxane), and vitamin D. Cholesterol further acts as an insulating bandage over abrasions and tears in the inner membrane of the arterial walls that get damaged because of the rush of "concentrated" pulsating blood, which becomes acidic and possibly corrosive when the body becomes dehydrated. What you see as cholesterol plaques in the arterial system of blood circulation has never been seen in the veins of the body. This simple explanation reveals that the reasons offered for pushing cholesterol-lowering medication on people in our commerce-driven society are based more on fraud than science!

- All the cells of the body can use fatty acids interchangeably with glucose for energy. Thus, if the body has no problem burning fat, why do we insist on giving it more carbohydrate than fat? Even brain cells, after a few weeks, can learn to derive up to 50 to 75 percent of their energy from fat instead of sugar.

- This is the reason the body stores 150 times more energy in the form of fat than in the form of glycogen (starch).

- For each 9.3 calories of excess energy, 1 gram of fat will be deposited in the fat stores.

- About one-third of energy in normal people goes into muscle activity. In physically active people, as much as three-fourths of the energy consumed could be used for maintaining muscle activity. Thus, physical activity that engages the main muscle mass in the body is the best way to tap into the energy reserves of the body stored in its fat deposits.

- The total amount of stored starch in the entire body that will get used up in dieting or starvation is around a few hundred grams—good for only about half a day. Fat and proteins follow suit, fat more quickly than proteins. But loss of proteins could be detrimental, particularly as some of the more vital essential amino acids get attacked and become depleted from the body because they get used as antioxidants.

- The onset of some serious diseases begins with the loss and depletion of the essential amino acids.

When muscles are inactive, their energy stores are more easily attacked, and even their protein reserves are ultimately broken down for conversion into sugar. However, if muscles are used, they begin to metabolize some of their stored fat as a choice source of energy to do work and maintain or increase their bulk. To do this, they begin to activate a fat-breaking enzyme called hormone-sensitive lipase. Repeated blood tests in a company of Swedish soldiers on a three weeks march showed that this enzyme's activity is seen after 1 hour's walk; it remains in circulation and retains its fat-breaking activity for 12 hours. The activity of the enzyme becomes cumulative with increased walking. The soldiers showed very strong activity of their hormone-sensitive lipase throughout their march.

Why is this information significant? As you know, the bulk of our bodies' muscle content is located in the legs and hips, the anatomical parts used in locomotion. Also significant is the fact that burning fat for locomotion is economical: One gram of fat provides more than twice as much energy for muscle activity as what the equivalent weight of sugar or protein provides. One gram of fat generates 9 calories of energy, whereas 1 gram of sugar or of protein provides

4 calories. Burning fat is the most efficient way for the muscles to use the body's energy stores. Thus, making and retaining fat is the most efficient way to establish an energy reserve for the body to be used at times of scarcity, such as in winter. This information alone indicates that we are wrong in reducing the fat in our diets; instead, we should eat more healthy oils and fat and less carbohydrate.

Water and Fat Storage

There is an inverse relationship between water consumption and fat accumulation in the body. The less water you drink, the more you will be forced to eat. The more you eat, unless you are physically active, the more you store fat. Here are the reasons:

- Water is the primary source of energy for all physiological functions of the body.

- Water turns "micro-electric turbines"—the cation pumps—and generates electricity for neurotransmission and nerve impulses in the entire body.

- Every food item that has to be broken down and metabolized will need the chemical influence of water—hydrolysis—before its energy can be utilized by the cells of the body. In effect, as was shown in the formula for magnesium-ATP, water transfers its hidden energy to the substances it breaks down—increasing their energy content by about one order of magnitude.

- In cell membranes, water is used for its stickiness—like the ice that sticks to your fingers—and acts as the adhesive that holds membrane structures together. In dehydration, the stickiness of cholesterol has to hold and insulate the cell membrane— hence we see a gradual rise in cholesterol levels from increased food intake when the body is dehydrated.

- The constant communication of nine trillion brain cells is energy-dependent and must be powered by either hydroelectric energy or energy from the metabolism of food. Excess energy from hydroelectricity is stored in the form of ATP, and the extra water leaves the body in the form of urine. It does not form a "lake" in the body. Excess energy from food taken to maintain brain activity is stored in the form of fat—only 20 percent of "solid" energy from food reaches the brain, while the rest is stored as fat, unless used in physical activity.

- The early sensation of thirst and sensation of hunger— stemming from low brain energy levels—are similar. They get reflected in heartburn/hunger pang sensations. We never recognized heartburn as an indicator of thirst until I treated 3,000 people suffering from the heartburn of peptic ulcer disease with only water; I later proved this sensation to mean thirst for water. We traditionally treated this sensation, before it became severe, as though it were only a hunger pain— hence overeating when the body is actually thirsty. This confusion is background to getting fat—we eat more food, even before full digestion of earlier meals, hence indigestion, gas formation, and bloating. Taking a glass of water before eating and allowing time for the satiety mechanism to kick in would correct this mistake. A glass of water will work more efficiently than any antacid or gas-reducing medication.

- Taking a glass of water before eating would also stimulate secretion of adrenaline and noradrenalin by the sympathetic system for at least two hours. This direct action of water on the sympathetic nervous system forcefully activates hormone-sensitive lipase to break down fat for use as energy to enhance the physical activity of the body. This is the reason water overrides the sensation of hunger in a short period of time.

- The human body recycles and constantly circulates around 40,000 glasses of water in every 24 hours (from information published by Loma Linda University in California). If each glass of water is 250 cubic centimeters or 8 ounces, then the circulation is hauling about 10,000 liters or 2,500 gallons of water every 24 hours. This physiological function is intensely energy consuming—hence the release of energy from the fat stores of the body through the sympathetic nervous system activation of lipase, when we drink water.

- Thus, water has two strong direct effects in preventing the body from becoming obese. First, by providing "clean" energy for brain function, it avoids the storage of fat from excess food intake. Second, by constantly activating the fat-burning enzymes, water tips the balance in favor of breaking up the fat reserves when the body is going through the process of recycling its fat stores. This is the reason people who choose the WaterCure lose weight without any effort.

- One advantage of adequate hydration for reducing the fat stores of the body is the fact that you don't need to count calories. Your taste buds and the satiety mechanism of your body will do the work for you.

- After you drink a glass of water, for up to two hours it will stimulate the secretion of one of the gut's dominant hormones, motilin. Motilin acts exactly like serotonin. Serotonin, in turn, is the chief of all neurotransmitters in the brain; it regulates all the brain's physiological responses to outside stimulation. Serotonin is what depressed people do not have enough of. They take medications to protect its presence in their bodies. Normal people have enough serotonin in their brains and nerve systems. When water stimulates the release of motilin, it in fact is causing the brain to know that water is on board and thirst is quenched. Motilin is a satiety hormone.

- Motilin does yet another thing: It activates motility in the intestines and promotes passage of their contents downstream. It acts as a laxative. Thus, two glasses of water first thing in the morning will be a more effective intestinal stimulant and a lubricating laxative than anything else you might imagine—and it is all natural and what the body wanted all the time. Your body will not need to squeeze the contents of its guts for their last drop of water, making what should be routine bowel movements painful events.

- The satiety action of motilin will overcome any sensation that you might interpret as a feeling of hunger. This is the reason people who want to diet and lose weight need to drink water before any food and give it time to override their perception of hunger. What's happening is simple: Water provides hydro-electric energy for the brain, and the low energy sensation of the brain that is commonly interpreted as "hunger" is canceled. At the same time lipase, activated by the sympathetic nervous system, will shunt the metabolic direction of the body into fat breakdown and its conversion into energy—the same ATP that you would make from sugar. "The quick fix with sugar" for the panic-stricken brain will not be needed until you drink your next glass or two of water.

- The regular intake of water will keep the physiology of your body in its fat-breaking mode until you take your next sugary or starchy food. They encourage insulin-induced fat storage and "hypoglycemic panics" that force you to eat more of the same. To overcome this problem, it is more prudent to eat protein snacks that might even be high in their fat content. Do not be frightened of some fat in your diet. It is not the fat content of your diet that causes heart disease. It is chronic unintentional dehydration—and its associated mineral deficiencies—that is the primary cause of heart problems.

- Remember, when your daily diet does not include adequate water, you do not properly absorb the minerals in your food. This is when the body becomes acidic, and acidic blood eats into the delicate arterial membranes. You need water and minerals to get rid of the acidic waste products of metabolism in the urine you pass out—the light color of urine is a good indicator of an alkaline body. Dark yellow or orange urine means an acidic body, the primary indicator of the onset of heart disease.

Water is a natural medication for people who tend to put on weight. To lose already gained weight, water is more effective than anything in the arsenal of the drug or diet industry. When you give water a chance to fulfill its primary role in bodily energy formation, your natural leanings for food will shift from starch to protein and fat, and your cravings for sugary stuff will be few and far between.

The next step would be to add muscle activity to enhance the action of water on the fat-breaking enzyme lipase. If you wish to lose weight as a crash course, two walking sessions—one in the morning and one in the evening—will activate lipase around the clock, even while you sleep. Not only will you begin to lose fat from your body, but you will also clear the cholesterol "bandage" from the acid-damaged walls in your arteries that can now get repaired—a welcome fringe benefit.

Fat stores in the body also collect some of the toxic chemicals that foods are sprayed or prepared with. When fat is released for energy, you need the extra water to wash out these released chemicals.

You have to pay attention to your minerals and salt intake to keep all the pumps active for hydroelectric energy formation. The last chapters of this book are devoted to a discussion of diet and minerals.

I suppose you'd now like to hear some reports on the effectiveness of proper hydration as a means of losing weight. Here are some success stories. As you'll see, when you correct the dehydration of the body, not only do you lose weight, but you also get rid of many other disease complications of dehydration.

Most of the people who lost 20, 30, or 40 pounds did not start the program of rehydration of their bodies to lose weight; they were focusing on their other health problems, such as asthma, hypertension, back pain, and more. They were not dieting to lose weight. Their weight loss was the natural outcome of hydrating their bodies.

And what of the people who were out to lose weight? Their loss was so impressive that it surprised everyone around them. They lost their excess pounds without hassle or too much effort. The kind of loss that was achieved with increased water intake is the kind for which some people undergo drastic, mutilating surgery. The long-term outcome of such operations is not yet known. One thing is sure, though: If there are problems ahead, unfortunately the surgery cannot be reversed.

The stomach has many, many functions other than just making you fat! Getting fat is a problem of willpower—but also of ignorance of the water's roles in metabolic processes. Stomach acid serves as a barrier against bacterial contaminants in food. It is vital for processing the minerals in the diet. It is vital for absorption of vitamin B12, which is indispensable in blood manufacturing processes. Shortage of vitamin B12 in the body can cause pernicious anemia. Lack of B12 can lead to spinal cord damage and can be responsible for paralysis of the lower extremities. I have seen this kind of sub-clinical B12 deficiency—which was not diagnosed by eminent physicians in California—cause paralysis of both legs in a young lady who ultimately died at a very early age because of the progressive complications of her disease. (At least she died rich; she was awarded punitive damages for misdiagnosis of her problems.) Having an intact stomach would prevent such complications.

You need the hydrochloric acid in the stomach to be able to absorb the essential minerals from your food. Magnesium, zinc, selenium, manganese, and others need to be "acid treated" in the stomach before they become absorbable. Only then can they be assimilated into the enzyme systems that need their presence to achieve potency.

You now understand the role of water in weight regulation. What you might need in addition is strong willpower to overcome the urge to feast on sweet stuff. All you need to do is to stand in front of the mirror and tell yourself you want to be slimmer than you are. Create an image of a smaller you in your mind, and revisit this image over and over again until your mind is made up. Your brain is a very sophisticated computer. It will begin to program its chemical demands and controls on the basis of the newly installed program in its subconscious mind. After you have made sure your brain knows a slimmer you is what you want, you will automatically avoid all the goodies you ate in the past. Make sure you give your body ample water, some vital minerals, and salt for their essential energy-making activities. It is my professional understanding that most overweight people are subconsciously compelled to overeat to obtain their sodium and other mineral needs. Unfortunately, they do not realize that they also need water to absorb these minerals.

TWO PEARLS TO ENRICH YOUR THOUGHTS:

- You need to prevent thirst to lose weight. When you wait to get thirsty to drink water, you get confused and think you are actually hungry, even if you ate only two or three hours ago. When you are fully hydrated, the constructive effect of food will last, and it will be a long time before you're hungry again. You should quench your thirst with water; manufactured and taste-enhanced beverages that are sweetened to make them marketable defeat the purpose and turn off the fat-burning enzymes.

- When you reduce your food intake and increase your water intake to lose weight, supplement your diet with vitamins and minerals. You must make sure you do not become deficient in those minerals, which you would normally get from your food. Also, be sure to use unrefined salt from the ocean or old salt mines in the mountains—not the regular table salt that is stripped of its companion minerals. Salt and mineral cravings force you to overeat.

SATIETY MECHANISMS

Fat tissue is also an endocrine gland. It produces many hormones. One of these is called lepitin. Leptin is supposed to let the brain know when the fat reserves are fully replenished. Obviously, in fat people, the mechanism is ineffective. I do believe proper hydration corrects this discrepancy between leptin levels in blood circulation and their proper assessment by the brain cells.

Another satiety mechanism is connected to the stretch sensors in the stomach. This is when the brain realizes enough is enough. The more we eat and force the stomach to stretch, the more the brain becomes insensitive to the message system from the stretch sensors in the stomach. The brain gets used to the over-stretching of the stomach tissue—this is the case with all fat people.

The most effective and least understood food intake control mechanism is attached to the taste buds on the tongue. This control system could only work when food is held in the mouth as long as possible while chewing it. The taste buds register with the brain the volume and type of food that has been processed and passed through. The slow rate of chewing—until the food is totally minced into very small particles, and even liquified by its mixing with saliva, gives the brain time to calculate the energy value of what has passed into the stomach—the satiety mechanism takes over and possible over eating will stop. Try it.

Stories That Lift Your Heart

Imagine having to sleep in an upright position for almost a year, struggling for each breath and suffering from countless asthma and panic attacks nightly! That was me until five months ago! On March 27, 1993, I was hospitalized with a severe asthma attack and developed bronchial pneumonia! My blood gases registered 40 and I was in a life-threatening situation!

After my release from the hospital, I was placed on large doses of theophylline and prednisone. My weight skyrocketed and the medication caused me to become hostile and disoriented. I really didn't want to live! Then, a wonderful friend gave me a flyer on Dr. Batmanghelidj's book Your Body's Many Cries for Water! I quickly mailed a check and a letter to the doctor, pleading for a fast delivery! To my complete surprise, he called me personally and started helping me by telephone to get off the medication, which was inappropriate for my condition at this time, and asked me to drink at least three liters of water a day and use a small amount of salt. He also asked me to walk in an indoor shopping mall for 15 minutes a day. I can now walk for 30 minuets a day and my breathing is 100% better!

As of this date, October 31, 1994, I am no longer on any medication for asthma! I have not used an inhaler or medication of any sort for more than five months! When I start any sort of mild wheezing, I just drink a glass of water and take a little salt and I'm fine!

And guess what???? All the wonderful water and walking has made me lose 35 lbs. I'm back to my desired weight and I look young, vibrant, and healthy again!

There are millions of Americans out there who need to get the message. They suffer from AIDS, asthma, arthritis, chronic fatigue syndrome, etc. Everyone in America could benefit from reading Dr. Batmanghelidj's books!

Very sincerely, P. P.

This letter is a testimony to the merits of water as an essential part of the daily dietary requirements for good health. I have been following your recommendations for nearly five years, and have found myself taking for granted the positive effects of water intake.

When I first started on the program I was overweight, with high blood pressure and suffering from asthma and allergies, which I have had since a small child. I had been receiving treatment for these conditions. Today, I have my weight and blood pressure under control (weight loss of approximately 30 pounds and a 10-point drop in blood pressure). The program reduced the frequency of asthma and allergy-related problems, to the point of practical nonexistence. Additionally, there were other benefits I experienced; fewer colds, flu, and generally with less severity.

I introduced this program to my wife, who had been on blood pressure medication for the past four years, and through increased water intake has recently been able to eliminate her medication.

Thanks again for your program, M. P.

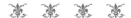

I again wish to thank you for your kindness in helping my wife and me to better appreciate the importance of water to our health.

We feel the conscious increase in our water consumption contributed greatly to our weight loss—a weight loss that had been urged upon both of us by our respective physicians for years. My loss of approximately 45 pounds has resulted in such a lowering of my blood pressure that I am no longer taking medications for my blood pressure. My wife's weight loss has alleviated the discomfort she has experienced for years with her back. In addition, she believes the weight loss has reduced her discomfort and problems with her allergies.

With best wishes, I remain

Sincerely, E. M. P.

Note: Dr. M. G. is a nutrition consultant. After reading my book, she convinced her daughter Donna to begin changing her fluid intake habits. The result has astounded both mother and daughter. The following is verbatim transcript of Donna's testimonial.

My mother asked that I write to you and tell you about my recent weight loss success. I know that I could have a much more successful loss if I would follow your formula and curb my eating habits, along with starting a regular routine of exercise. However just getting myself to get off of 6 to 8 cans of Mountain Dew a day is a miracle in itself.

Within the last 9 months to a year, I have successfully been able to keep 35 excess pounds of baggage off. I am able to wear clothes that I thought would never touch my body again. I also have just about reached my goal size for my upcoming wedding. Even my fiancé had to admit that I am looking much better than when he first met me five years ago.

My success has been contributed to faithfully drinking half my body weight in ounces in water every day. Wherever I go, so does my water. To work, shopping, even my long 7-hour-long car rides. (That does make for a lot of rest area stops, but they are worth it.) I do treat myself to an occasional mineral water or beer when I go out, but I have usually gotten my quota of water in for the day.

One interesting thing that I have noticed however is that once I have finished drinking my quota of water, I have absolutely no desire to drink anymore. Also I have found that I'm not thirsty anymore and it will usually take me a while to drink some other type of beverage whether it be juice, milk, beer, mineral water, etc.

I am looking forward to October 1, which is my wedding day when I can walk down the aisle looking better than I have looked in 15 years, since I graduated from high school. It will also be nice to put my weight on my new driver's license without having to cringe for the first time in my life.

Thanks for the smaller me!!!! Donna M. G.

Dear Dr. Batmanghelidj:

In November of 2000, I weighed 525 lbs. Now, January of 2003, I weigh 225. Here is how I did it.

My story is simple. For thirty-two years of my life I continued to eat all the wrong foods and drink every unhealthy drink imaginable. My life for thirty-two years was a happy one. I had lots of friends, good jobs, and a wonderful, but sickly mother. I got around pretty well for someone of my size. I was active, playing sports and competing in karate, all such activities that would promote a healthy lifestyle or weight loss. I however ate everything that was bad for you in large amounts, at the wrong times, and would follow it up by drinking liters of soda or alcohol.

I look back now and could honestly say without any reservation that there were times of up to a month that I would not have any water. Water never tasted good to me, and as far as could remember, it would always give me a stomachache. Maybe it did. Maybe it was psychological, because I really didn't need or want to drink water. I loved soda and could easily sit and drink a two-liter bottle with one meal. One meal could be a large pizza with everything and chicken wings, 10:30 at night. I could recall two to three times a week I would order from a local pizza place a large cheese steak with extra cheese and a meatball with extra cheese and eat both with a two-liter soda, again very late at night. The times I remember eating the most was when I was alone at night or just getting home from work late at night, not tired, and would eat. Even at the times when I wasn't really hungry. It became routine for me to do this regularly.

My mornings weren't the best either. I made daily stops to the local McDonald's on my way to work to order two to three breakfast sandwiches and again my favorite soda. Looking back now I realized this routine went on for years to the point I couldn't say honestly when I started this massive destruction of my body. It didn't help to have a few friends who were also big people who ate a lot. My friends and I would regularly hit every buffet in the city. It got to the point where we were recognized and our names called out like Norm on Cheers. Not something to be proud of. Earlier on I stated I was a very happy person and had many wonderful friends. However I was very lonely; I had no one to share myself with.

Just about all of my friends were married, in love, and had beautiful companions to come home to. Everything I always wanted for myself but was not realistic at my size. Losing weight was not believable to me. My mother was very ill, in and out of the hospital multiple times with lung disease. A few times she almost didn't make it. I was very scared and again found another excuse to eat and eat a lot. My mother did eventually get a little better and didn't need me there all the time.

In November of 2000, at the age of thirty, I started seriously considering stomach stapling to help me lose weight, if I wanted to honestly live. At that weight the chances of living much longer wouldn't be too good. I was feeling the stress of my massive weight on all my joints, was getting ill more often, and was hospitalized multiple times with deep vein thrombosis. I was very scared and very alone. I knew it was time to get serious about losing weight or die. I guess you're wondering how much I weighed. I weighed a whopping 525 lbs. I wore a six-extra-large shirt and had a waistline of seventy-two. On January 21 of 2001 I started my very long journey to a new life.

I had a very good friend who pushed me nightly for three months straight to go with him to the gym and eat the right foods at the right times. Most importantly drink a lot of water. I mean a lot of water. I hated water, but I knew if I really wanted to lose weight I needed to do the right thing and stop playing games. At this time for the first time in my life I was confident about myself and knew I had it in me to lose any amount of weight I needed to. I met a wonderful woman at about the same time I began my journey to become healthy and hopefully thin. My friend pushed me harder and was always there for me not to give up. I made up my mind to give up all liquids besides water and a popular diet drink. It helped me a lot. I would wake up every morning and have a diet drink and drink a 24-oz glass of water. I would drink three more 24-oz glasses of water before lunch, have another diet drink, and continue with my regimen of water until dinner. I would drink a 24-oz glass of water leading up to dinner to help me feel full and not want to eat as much.

I became very drastic with my eating habits and food. I would never eat past six o'clock at night and again only water to help me feel full. Let me tell you, I went to the bathroom all the time. I gave up all breads, pasta, and potatoes, everything that had carbohydrate in it. Most importantly I gave up all soda, even diet decaffeinated. My carbohydrate intake was about twenty grams a day and my saturated fat intake was about two to three grams a day. I know you're saying that your body needs fat to survive. You are absolutely right. I was prepared during my weight loss in what is healthy and what isn't while dieting. I read and read multiple books on vitamins and supplements to make sure I wasn't depriving my body of what it needed. I also saw a doctor regularly. I began taking daily essential fatty acids in pill form along with a multivitamin, a vitamin B complex 150, calcium, vitamin C, and a sublingual vitamin B12. All of which, I learned, help with energy metabolism and the breakdown of stored fat, carbohydrates, and sugar.

A great person, and now great friend, who owned a local fitness store broke it down for me honestly and helped me with my supplement regiment. My nightly cardiovascular and weight routine began to get easier as I began losing weight fast. I was almost losing a pound of weight a day. People were getting worried but I remained true to eating the right foods and drinking the huge amounts of water. My doctor continued to monitor me and was not too concerned with my rapid weight loss. My blood pressure was getting better along with my resting heart rate lowering and, thank God, no problems with sugar diabetes.

I guess you are wondering what I was eating. Well, I was eating large amounts of canned tuna and canned chicken. Protein, protein, and protein, as much as I could get, lots of salad with no dressing, turkey burgers, vegetable burgers, and again lots and lots of chicken and tuna. Yes, I was sick of eating the same thing all the time. However, I kept reminding myself the diet and exercise was working and I was losing weight. I encouraged myself to believe that pasta, pizza, soda, cheeseburgers, and other junk weren't more important to me than my life. Oh yes, let me tell you of the wonderful woman I mentioned briefly earlier on. I continued to see her and her two beautiful boys. This was more motivation to continue than anything anyone could imagine. I was in love and most importantly someone was in love with me. Yes, she fell in love with the fat me, which makes her even more special to me.

As the months went on I continued ever diligently on my exercise and water regimen. I never felt sick and I never again had any problems with the veins in my legs. People were beginning to notice the change that was occurring. It was getting drastic. My waistline was falling along with my shirt size. In case you forgot I weighed 525 lbs. At the end of the first year of my dieting, January 21, 2002, I weighed 250 lbs. I lost 275 lbs working very hard with friends and on my own. My current weight today, as of the New Year 2003, is 225 lbs. I found that this is a very good weight for me. I have put on good muscle and shrunk down to a large shirt and a 38 waist comfortably. I do have a lot of skin but hope to eventually get surgery to have it removed. A lot of skin from a lot of fat is a good trade-off to me.

Keeping the weight off is easy to me now that I have tons of energy, can get around—and running on the treadmill up to three miles at a time surely helps a lot. Yes, I currently eat all the foods I used to eat. Cheeseburgers, pizza, pasta, potatoes, and occasionally some candy. It's all about one word, moderation. Never ever again I will drink soda. Water . . . Water . . . Water . . . (Okay, diet green tea and a diet drinks.) Is all the weight loss real to me? I still don't believe it sometimes. When I look into a mirror there are times I don't believe it's me.

The first real time I knew I was actually thin and not fat is when I walked in front of a group of little kids going to school. None of them stared at me, or laughed, or made a fat comment. I had just passed the little-kid test. During my years of being fat I knew that kids were the toughest and most honest. My life today is everything I had dreamed about. Well, it's no longer a dream. I have married the woman I spoke

about and became a father to her two wonderful boys. Today we live a
beautiful life in a beautiful home with a very happy and healthy life. If
there is anything I can say to help anyone who reads this story, it is to
never give up. Dreams can be reality. Follow good advice and do it for
you. There is a famous quote that I kept in my wallet through my diet-
ing and still remains there today. Martin Luther King stated, "We
must accept finite difficulties, but we must never lose infinite hope." I
HAVEN'T AND NEVER WILL!

I am attaching my pictures before and after weight loss.

David Caruso

Note: If a picture is equal to a thousand words, the photos that follow speak volumes. The first thing that you can see—more than
the words in David's story could convey—is the fact that water is a
powerful medication for obese people. The second point these pictures make is the simplicity of using water to prevent getting fat,
provided staying slim is a marker of beauty in your mind. The third
thought would be: If only children in America could stop drinking
sodas and stick to water, what a healthy nation they would make
out of America—as simply as these words are written.

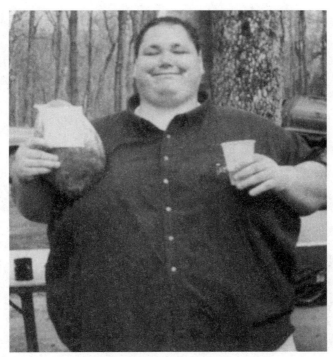

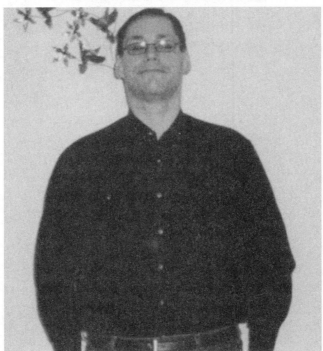

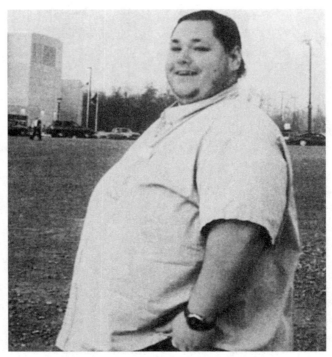

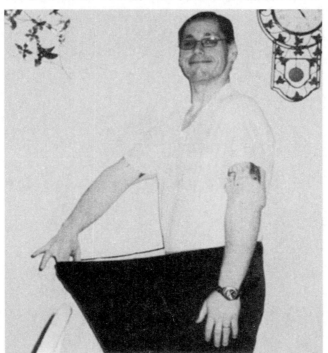

While waiting in line to pay for my groceries at the local supermarket, I suddenly noticed the following headline on the cover of Woman's World Magazine. I was shocked to see the topic of my interest was given such a prominent position in the magazine. I had absolutely no idea how this information had gotten into the magazine, and since I am used to other people taking my research and embellishing it as their own "reinvention of the wheel," I became curious to know who was being quoted and who had penned the article. Here is the text of the cover:

Woman's World Magazine
September 4, 2001

"She lost 30 lbs without dieting!" Revolutionary Medical Breakthrough:
The Slimming new Water Cure!

Learn how to <u>Drink</u> away 40 lbs or more! Finola Hughes of All My Children (picture on the cover)

The inside pages had a number of pictures and the headline:

"The 'Water Cure' can make you thin!"

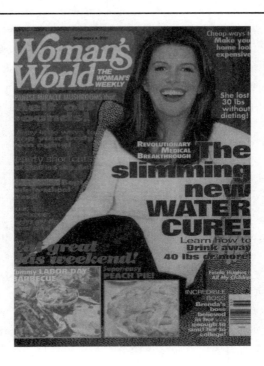

We can't rave enough about the latest
weight-loss breakthrough. It's simple,
safe, and effective. This M.D.-devised
technique has already worked wonders
for All My Children's Finola Hughes,
who shed 30 lbs. three times faster than
average— and without dieting. Read on
to discover how you can drink away as
much as 40 lbs. easily!

After reading these lines, I became more curious and started to scan the article. When I saw my own name and the title of my book *Your Body's Many Cries for Water*, I was extremely surprised and relieved. Apparently Ms. Hughes, who had lost 30 easy pounds without dieting, and could now fit into her better clothes looking elegant and trim, must have talked about my book and how she lost weight without dieting, creating interest in introducing my book to the readers of Woman's World Magazine. Also mentioned in the article was Amy Biank, a radio personality in the Chicago area. In six weeks she had reduced her size 20 measurements to a size 14, then a size 12. "At the time, I was getting out of bed in the morning feeling old and heavy," recalls the 54-year-old, who had been steadily gaining weight since her early 40s. "My joints ached. I would get overwhelmingly tired. I had hot flashes. . . ." "Amy has lost the weight, quadrupled her energy, eliminated achy joints, beaten her allergies and chased away menopause symptoms simply by drinking water—more specifically a doctor-prescribed amount of water," wrote the magazine.

If you get the chance to go to the library and find the magazine, the article might prove interesting reading. What I have stressed before, and what the above article highlighted, is the fact that with the WaterCure program, strict dieting is not necessary. You do not need to count calories, as in all the other diet programs. Your naturally selective food cravings will direct you to the foods your body needs. All you have to do is control your sweet tooth until the selective processes of your brain establish dominance and control. After that you will automatically avoid things that are not good for your figure.

Some More Impressive Results

Dear Dr. Batmanghelidj,

My wife and I have been following your water program for about 18 months. While we have always been in good health, we are certain that your discovery has no doubt added years and quality to our lives. We have also had two obvious benefits and without any real effort. My wife took off over 30 lbs. And she called it a breeze, especially since she tried weight loss programs before which were always a form of punishment and deprivation. I also took off 15 lbs and found the same. The unique thing about it is that we eat what we want, but aren't nearly as hungry, especially when we always drink a glass or two of water before eating. We can honestly say that you have made losing weight an easy thing to do.

Another thing is that I've had a bad back for nearly thirty years. Any time that I helped out in the warehouse where prolonged lifting was involved, I would limp around for several days while experiencing considerable pain, especially late that same day and the following day. While my back didn't become miraculously healed in a few weeks or a couple of months as I had seen happen to some of my friends, it did become 99% healed in about 15 months and I can do everything that I could do before my injury without pain. To me, that's incredible.

I have passed information on to countless people as I found that many had miraculous health benefits in a matter of days. Your discovery has impressed me to the point that my company has told tens of thousands of your discovery by running thousands of newspaper ads (some full page), television ads, and radio ads to get the word out. Radio spots alone now number over 400 a month. Many of our customers who were in their early sixties, were getting out of their business because of problems of health and age only to be planning to renew their efforts and some even expanding their business after a few weeks of your program.

Without a doubt, I could write a book on what I've seen. I told everyone who has been helped in any way that I hoped they would feel a moral responsibility to pass this information on to at least ten people who also gain a considerable health improvement.

This effort has resulted in various interviews and we even helped form a foundation called "The Circle of Light" to help improve the quality of life in northeastern PA in the areas of health, human relations, and education. I have spoken to many doctors who have called for information and even interviewed two on a radio program who have stated that they make your water program part of their treatment.

The truth of your work has caught me up with an incredible passion that will not diminish until the most of our country accepts what you have done as just common sense. I sincerely thank you for providing me the opportunity of a lifetime in extremely positive public service. Thanks to you Dr. Batmanghelidj, tens of thousands of people in northeastern PA have had their lives improved.

Sincerely yours, Bob Butts

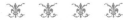

I was drinking two or more pots of coffee and a few sodas every day. No water. I am retired about three years now, while working I would drink some water from the cooler at work. Now that I am home I don't have a cooler and don't like tap water so I drank none at all.

SYMPTOMS:

My urine was getting very strong. I thought I would need to see a doctor soon for a possible infection.

My constipation was so bad I was using hemorrhoid preparation 2 to 3 times a week. My stomach burned sometimes so I used Tums a few times a month. Also I seemed to have some sort of bronchial problem, a deep cough, soreness, and very thick phlegm.

During the winter it was necessary to wear long johns for the first time in my life. At night I needed socks, long johns, and a T-shirt and I would cover up with a sheet and two blankets. I was so cold in the morning I would use a blow dryer to warm my feet, then after putting socks on I would warm the socks on my feet. Lastly, I would heat the shoes I was going to wear. It was common to be cold enough I could hardly function. It was painful.

If I tried to go for a walk I would wear two pairs of gym pants. I went to the gym and used the treadmill and cross-trainer. I started feeling depressed when I got to the gym, didn't know why. My numbers had been slowly decreasing—that is, the speed and inclination settings. I always hold the sides.

When I walked freely at the shopping mall my sides would hurt so badly it brought me to tears. My feet would hurt but the side pain overwhelmed this.

My karate lessons have been getting harder and harder. The number of moves, like kicks, I could do has been dropping regularly. The instructor wanted 25 to 50 kicks and we have been reducing this to 10 to 15, kept saying I was getting old disregarding how fast I was aging in just a few years.

I had been trying to lose weight but if I cut back my food intake I would get cold and achy much like getting a cold. I was getting so uncomfortable I did not like to get up in the morning, just didn't feel good to sit or stand. I can understand how lack of enthusiasm or lethargy or even depression could set in.

One curious thing I noticed was on the skin of my hand. When I held my hand out the skin seemed like mummy skin, very dry. My hand was flat.

I was starting to worry about my health, maybe diabetes. I have always tested fine for this, and my Web research did not seem to support anything I could find.

I know doctors tell you to drink water when ill, so the strong urine caused me to start drinking water to flush my system. About the same time a friend sent me an e-mail about dehydration. I was shocked to learn a few percent dehydration could cause a 10 to 20 percent drop in athletic output. This e-mail led me to do research on the Web. I was amazed to find I had almost all of the signs of dehydration. I decided to look for books and eventually found your book, Your Body's Many Cries for Water at Amazon. I have been following the regime of 2 or more glasses first thing in the morning, one one-half hour before each meal, one 2 and a half hours after each meal, and one at night. During the day I drink a little more, a glass or two. Also the coffee intake has been reduced.

RESULTS:

- *My urine no longer smells and the constipation has almost completely disappeared.*

- *I didn't know bowel movements were this easy, it's almost pleasant.*

- *My stomach is fine now and the bronchial discomfort is gone.*

- *I now sleep in just underwear just like years ago. I have had many nights when my legs felt so warm they almost felt sweaty. It's amazing how far off my body's temperature regulation had gotten. When I am exposed to cold it just feels cold, it doesn't hurt anymore.*

- *When I get up in the morning I feel fine. Sometimes I just enjoy sitting because I feel so good, no discomfort. When I drink 2 or 3 glasses when I first get up I get a lift from it similar to what we get from coffee. If I go on the computer in the morning the screen is brighter, seems to sparkle. I don't understand this but it happens.*

- *When I cut back on my eating to lose weight I just get hungry, not sick. I actually smile at this because I feel I have control. A little hunger but I can stand it.*

- *Regarding my hand. Now when I hold my hand out the blood vessels show and there are little muscle bumps all over. Before my hand was flat. I never feel depressed anymore. I attribute this to just feeling better. Slight pain and/or discomfort slowly grinds away at one's attitude.*

- *Some problems slowly sneak up on a person and we don't notice the degradation or we adapt to it. The most directly measurable result is at the gym. Using the same speed and elevation settings as before my heart is 10 to 12 points lower. At first I thought this was the machine but all the equipment shows this.*

Some of these fixes occurred very quickly, a few days; some took a month or two to completely take effect.

Overall, I am amazed at the influence of low water intake. I have clear-cut results and much optimism. My karate instructor now wants me to get my Black Belt. This seems amazing to do at 60 but I did have training in my 20s. He is sure I can do it, and the system I am studying does not give the belts out easily like some do. This makes me feel very proud and has increased my self-esteem. It makes me want to do more things.

I read and reread your book often. Many of the things in your book I would not even believe a few months ago but I have proof. I highly recommend the book to everyone I know. I have become a water spokesman. There seem to be many examples among my friends, especially the older ones. There are people over 50 that drink nothing but coffee, tea, or alcohol and they have most of the symptoms I had. If I can just get them to cut back the coffee and drink water I am happy and feel I am helping. It is easy to imagine how dehydration can lead to serious disease. My informal data gathering seems to indicate a serious dehydration problem with the elderly, especially older men.

It is very clear your book is very valuable. My only criticism is I had to reread to find your daily routine for water consumption, wish you had this as a separate chapter or table.

There is no question your book is a valuable service to an important topic, thank you very, very much. I also enjoyed your discussion on diet beverages though this was not one of my problems. As a matter of fact, the book is a must read, far more valuable for good health than possibly anything else on the shelf.

In one of the letters from readers of your book it was said he kept two books on his nightstand. The Bible and yours. At first I thought this was funny but you know what, your book may be that important. It has improved the quality of my life.

Paul C. V.-K.

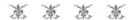

My many thanks for your research and wonderful book, Your Body's Many Cries for Water.

The commonsense approach to health certainly works. In the past eight weeks I have changed my eating and drinking lifestyle. At 53 it is wonderful to have lost 25 lbs., a lean and fit 6 feet, 181 lbs., and I ran 2.5 miles this morning. Water has played a great part in this transformation, not only the drinking but having a high water-content diet. What is really great is that my dust mite allergy for which I previously took a daily nasal spray has gone—no spray for eight weeks. We even slept without all the special covers on the bed last night!

I can assure you that I will continue to keep your ripple spreading.

Yours, R. W.

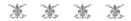

I am a Registered Nurse. I have been trained to think in terms of drugs for a long time. Drug reps are frequent visitors and educators with CEU info. I have also for over 10 years had to take Zantac, Prilosec, Prevacid, Maalox, and Gaviscon on a daily basis. I read The ABC of Asthma, Allergies, and Lupus and have to admit I was very skeptical. However, the thing that intrigued me was that there can't possibly be any monetary reason to shift someone into a water regimen. There is just no money in it. I also was getting a bit desperate, since in spite of everything, the medication wasn't working. My doctor was talking of a surgery that would cut nerves in my stomach to reduce the acid production. I am not thrilled with this type of permanent mutilation.

I decided to give water a try. It has been nearly two weeks since I decided to give it a try. I have not had any drugs since. As a bonus, my fall allergies have gone away. I am absolutely stunned. I also am sharing it with my patients. I also used to find it very difficult to stick to a diet and have had a lot of trouble losing weight. Not anymore. I have lost 5 pounds in 10 days and feel it much easier to say no to snacks. I just wish more people knew about this.

Thank you, Dean

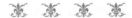

I want you to know how much I appreciate your "WaterCure," share this testimonial to help others make healthier lifestyle changes—your book has changed my life forever! Thank you!

In August of 1995, at age fifty, I found myself approaching 400 pounds. I swore to myself I would never hit 400. Life became a very painful experience. Every move I made was a painful episode as I struggled to survive. I also began having arthritic pains in my joints; so much that just shaking someone's hand was an unbelievably painful experience. Topping it off was a slipped disc in my back, so you can imagine just getting out of bed was a major effort.

I began getting depressed and irritated. I would find more things wrong than right with others and myself. At that point, I hit my pain threshold and that's when I came across a radio program with your message on wellness with water. Thank God for hearing this message. I heard about your book on that program and decided to read it. After reading it I decided to make some drastic changes in my life, which I did. My weight leveled off at 399 pounds. Then it started dropping. The more I drank *water and ate salt, the better I felt and the better I looked. I lost a total of 156 pounds and reduced 14 pant sizes. And I did this by drinking the amount of water you recommend, using table salt, and walking.*

Since losing the weight, I no longer have the stress on my joints and my back feels great. If you told me a year ago that I could feel this great, I would have said you're crazy, but it worked and I am living proof. I find myself telling everyone I can about your book and the greatest health discovery in history! I hope this letter will help others to try your cure, water and salt. It makes so much sense and it's so simple. I hope people will just try if for their own health's sake instead of becoming addicted to every medicine out there. Thank you very much for your discovery!!!

Sincerely, L. D.

🎖   🎖   🎖   🎖

For some time now, I have been trying to write to you to inform you of my progress using your system of the WaterCure. As you know, I seriously started your program back in 1997.

I lost 30 pounds in 31 days, lost all symptoms of my 19 years of asthma, allergies, and bronchitis as well as lost all desire for alcohol. I remember people telling me how my skin "glowed," which was in itself a miracle because I had such bad acne not only on my face, but also on my shoulders, back, and arms. On top of all that, I had arthritis on my hands. It was especially hard to decorate cakes and cookies, which I did professionally, because of the pain. I no longer have that problem either.

Now let me do a breakdown. I weighed approx. 192 pounds. And I am 5 feet, 4 inches tall. Or shall I say that is how short I am. I am now down to and remaining steady at 160 (give or take a few pounds because of the holidays) I can now fit into clothes I never was able to get in but I knew I would one day. You can't imagine how great it feels to have my kids and others call me "skinny" instead of the Crisco Kid—fat in the can! But the best feeling is when Bob holds me and his arms fit all around me now and then some.

When I first met you, I had allergies that were so bad that my eyes would swell up each and every morning. They itched so unbearably that I became addicted to an eye cream that the doctors had given me. Instead of drinking the iced tea, you told me to put it on my eyes and it worked. I stopped drinking all caffeine at that point but I was not able to give up the beer at that time. That came later. I had bronchitis twice a year, which was devastating. I could count on having an attack when the seasons changed from summer to fall and winter into spring. I'm sure my doctor has probably given me up for dead, because I have not had to call him in years for the antibiotic and cough medicine.

Just this past Thanksgiving, someone asked me if I were using a special lotion for my face because I looked younger.

With all the problems I had in the past, I know that it is difficult to explain to someone that the simplicity of it all, is hydration as well as nutrition, but it is.

I will be eternally grateful for your discovery and all your help Dr. Batman. May God be with us all in spreading this discovery.

Healing Hugs, Connie G.

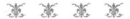

For most of my life, I have been overweight. Every family has a "fat child" and this was me. I was told that I was just "big boned" and I should be content with who I was. Then I heard about the water cure through Bob Butts and Connie Giblin. I was skeptical at first, because how could drinking iced tea and cola be such a problem. But I thought that all I really had to lose was my weight. Over a period of a year and a half, I have lost approximately 100 pounds and am no longer the "fat kid" that everyone knew.

But besides losing the weight, I have noticed that acid reflux, which had been a major part of my life, was also now gone; I could now enjoy foods that previously had brought me nothing but sickness. I have also noticed that I also no longer get ear infections that also seemed commonplace and inevitable problems of life to me at one time.

I also have more energy and feel as if I have become a whole new person. I have energy to do things that would easily wear me out previously.

Thank you Dr. Batman for helping me!

Sincerely, Mark C.

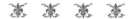

Hi, I am currently using the WaterCure to speed up weight loss. It was suggested on a low-carb bulletin board for friends of the Atkins way of eating. Just wanted you to know that right now I don't even care if it helps with weight loss, I feel so much better after only 6 days on WaterCure. My stress-related eczema is clearing up, my skin feels good, and even my hair feels great. A lot of the other Atkins friends are reporting benefits from WaterCure along with weight loss.

Thanks for listening. Pamela.

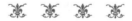

Dear Dr., I am a 100% total and perm. disabled vet, and have severe cervical pain from war injuries. I have been on morphine now for 7 years, and Dr. John Baranoski, N.D. (he and my daughter have just opened a day spa in Bar Harbor Maine), is trying to detox. me as much as I can.

My spine looks like the photos of a moose antlers, so not much can be done. But we are trying. While my daughter attended the Phoenix College of massage therapy, my wife of 32 years and myself babysat, and now that they have their business opened, they also have a copy of your book Your Body's Many Cries for Water on the front desk. I took to reading it and could not believe what I was reading. I quit soda two months ago as our trailer was broken into and $30,000 *damage was done. I felt so invaded that I thought an alarm would be better than the soda, so I quit.*

I lost 33 lbs in two months as a result, and the only downside was I had to buy new clothes. Not really a downside at all, it's just that on my pension we don't get much to live on, and have to be careful. But I do drink vast amounts of water and always have. Every time I was in the hospital, and that was many times, I was checked for sugar as I drank so much. I always have, and now even more. I want to thank you for writing the fine book I read and when I can afford more I will get them.

I want so bad to obtain good health as I always had until Vietnam, and then the tide changed a lot. I want to thank you for writing your books and want to add that as I progress I will keep you informed if you would like. I intend to deter as much as possible, but there was a great deal of damage done, and nothing can be done as there was years of no treatment or tests until I moved to Arizona where they treated me as a man not an animal. Sorry to be so frank but sometimes my feelings get away with me, and I won't say less than I feel.

Have a good day and I will if you wish keep in contact as wellness is my only true goal in life now and my wife of 32 years is a cert. herbalist, so as you can see my whole family is concerned with my getting better. That alone is a great boost in living a normal life.

Thank you very much. B. L. & P. L.

❦ ❦ ❦ ❦

Thank you for forwarding the information regarding AIDS as a metabolic disorder from the Science in Medicine Simplified Journal.

During the past year I have experienced many stressful life situations and have decided to look more seriously at my health and the care of my body. I have also started a master's degree in Wellness Science to further my knowledge for myself and for sharing with others. One of the most interesting and important subjects and one of your favorites is water, along with exercise and proper protein intake.

As I progress through my studies and begin to incorporate this new info and knowledge, I am finding a general overall increased well-being. I have more energy, stamina, sleep better, feel more peaceful, lost weight, and am beginning to see a difference in the edema swelling in my legs.

I am very appreciative for all that you share and I am daily sharing with others the importance of water and the other information that you so adequately shared in your book and related references.

Thank you kindly and you can rest assured that I am doing my utmost in educating the public about the importance of water.

Warmest regards, Janey P.

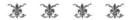

Hello!

What you're doing is absolutely fantastic, please don't ever stop!

The funny thing is—the WaterCure is so blindingly obvious that it is amazing we have to be told about it . . . but we do!

I run a business and was suffering from extreme tiredness, acne, and, due to all the sitting down in my office, was piling on the pounds. I put all of that down to the hard work of starting the business. Our kettle is the most overused piece of equipment in the office and I was drinking up to 8 cups a day.

As soon as I read about the WaterCure, I went out and bought a liter of mineral water. It took a while to wean myself off the tea but now, if I fancy a cup, it's always decaf. Within 1 month of drinking 1.5–3 liters of water a day, I have had to go and buy a new wardrobe of clothes, as all my old ones are falling off me! I have gone down 2 dress sizes! I have 100% more energy and concentration. My skin is clear and glowing!

I know a couple of people who are always complaining they can't shift weight—one of them has eczema and I know they drink a lot of tea. The other day, I said to them: if I could give you a tonic that would give you more energy, make your skin glow, make you lose weight and clear up your eczema, and on top of all that is completely free—would you take it? Oh yes, they said, definitely. I told them about the WaterCure and they said oh, no, I don't like water! Ah well, can't win them all!!

I can't thank you enough for what you are doing. Let us hope the message spreads far and wide.

P. M., United Kingdom

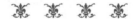

Thanks for your site.

In the past 3 months I have been drinking 3–4 liters of water a day and have shed approximately 30 pounds with no effort. I am certainly not starving myself but am eating healthy foods as a rule. (I still eat the occasional order of burgers, fries, and onion rings!) . . . the increase in energy I have felt has given me the ability to exercise, without pain, daily. And yes, I still have an occasional "pop"—but not 2 or 3 a day . . . Perhaps one per week . . . it has all been way too easy!!!

Water is truly what the body needs for good physical health . . .

Sincerely, N. A., Minnesota

After about ten days of the water and salt I feel fantastic. I also quit sugar and coffee and it really helps. I am losing my big belly so rapidly my pants are falling off of me. Thanks for sharing and caring.
Our E.A.P. specialist has been on the water program for about seven weeks. He weighed in at 295; he's presently lost 40 pounds; he's lost all traces of diabetes; his asthma has been noticeably relieved, and his skin has improved.

He now plays golf without back pain, and incidentally, this is very important to him. He's the biggest enthusiast we have and, as you know, as an E.A.P. specialist he's in the field contacting the people covered by our Insurance Trust daily, in that his specialty is drug addiction and alcoholism. He's taken many of our tapes, quite a few of our books, and is promoting the program personally.

I've been on the program for quite a while, and I feel that my indigestion has improved, my taste far more precise, and overall I feel it is working.

The same situation holds true for Phil Grisafi, our insurance manager, a young guy in his thirties, and to my knowledge, he's very, very, pleased with the results of the WaterCure so far. Will keep you posted. Once again, thank you for all your efforts and dedication.

⚜ ⚜ ⚜ ⚜

In 1995, I suffered a severe spinal injury playing football. I had used to live on caffeine drinks like soda, coffee, and teas. I turned to GOD and prayed! Then Dr. Su in Peckville, PA, put me on the WaterCure and I quit caffeine. The results? Fantastic energy! I lost 100 pounds.

In 5 1/2 months I was able to get off the 35 pills a day I was taking and all the above symptoms left. I used judo and jujitsu to work out and placed second in a national grappling competition.

My mom says, "We've been blessed with a miracle! I can't thank Dr. Su enough for the time and compassion he gave my son. He got his life back. And thanks to Dr. Batmanghelidj for bringing the WaterCure to the world."

Matt.

⚜ ⚜ ⚜ ⚜

First thanks for the tapes and reading material. Well we have been on the water/salt for 3 months now. Yes, there have been changes, subtle

*at first but now evident. For example, Janet and I lost 3 and 4 kilos
respectively (each kilo is 2.2 lbs).*

*Janet now has her dimples in her cheeks again. They have not been
evident for several years. We are both feeling lighter and more alive
inside ourselves. We are coping with some added pressures a lot better
than we would normally have done. Janet is now walking every second
day for about 3 kilometers, without feeling knocked out.*

*We shared this concept of water and salt with one of our daughters.
She has been taking Evening Primrose for some time now for tender
breasts. She stopped the tablets and has been on the water for 7 days.
No soreness, a feeling of life has returned. She has passed the message
onto another of our daughters and we will see what will happen.*

*Thanks to the good doctor and thanks to yourself for taking the mes-
sage to the people. Stay happy and keep up the great work.*

🎔 🎔 🎔 🎔

Note: In the following letter, you will see how simply a balanced
daily water intake also balances so many other important factors
that indicate better health, including the loss of 52 pounds.

*On February 12 my doctor called me with the results of my blood test
and informed me that I had Diabetes 2, as my Hemoglobin ALC was
7.3 and I weighed 348 lbs. The next day I started the WaterCure,
drinking 5 1/2 qts of water and adding 1 1/2 tsp. of salt to my food. I
just had my latest blood test on July 2, and here are the results.*

	02/12/02	07/02/02
Weight	348	296
Triglycerides	288	138
Cholesterol	247	189
Glucose	191	108
Hemoglobin ALC	7.3	5.4

I wasn't able to exercise during this time due to a bad back. So these results were achieved through the water and salt program. I eat all the normal foods. I am now starting to introduce an exercise routine using Dr. B.'s book for backs and can't wait to see the results. I would have never been able to get to this point without the water and salt and am eternally grateful to you and Dr. B. I now tell everyone I know about the water cure. Many thanks.

Thank you, John K.

OBESITY: THE HARBINGER OF DIABETES

Let me explain the relationship of dehydration to diabetes. The pancreas has a lot to do with water distribution in the body. You need to understand the mechanisms involved to realize why most obese people ultimately become diabetics, too.

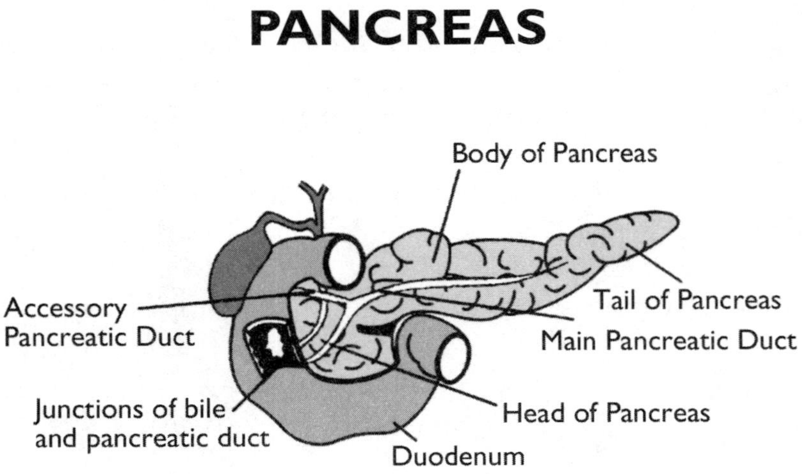

PANCREAS

Body of Pancreas

Accessory Pancreatic Duct

Tail of Pancreas

Main Pancreatic Duct

Junctions of bile and pancreatic duct

Head of Pancreas

Duodenum

Figure 4-1. The pancreas is positioned between the stomach and the first part of the small intestine. It produces insulin and the enzymes to digest the food components that enter the intestine.

The pancreas is situated such that its enzymes and bicarbonate solution can be injected into the intestine just as the acidic content of the stomach enters the intestine. The alkaline watery solution produced by the pancreas is designed to properly hydrate whatever enters the intestine, and to make the environment alkaline for the second phase of food digestion in the intestine. Whereas the contents of the stomach have to be acid, the contents of intestine must be alkaline and very liquid. The contents of the stomach are only released into the intestine when the pancreas is able to neutralize the acid and provide the water needed to microdigest food.

Many islands of cells in the pancreas, called beta-cells, produce insulin and release it into the circulation. The role of insulin is to open its "food gates" on the cell membranes of the body. When the body is optimally hydrated and is receiving all the components of food, insulin-sensitive receptors open up and sugar and amino acids can enter the cells, carrying the water needed for their cellular digestion with them.

Eating more food and drinking less water to the extent of obesity is very stressful to the pancreas. This organ initially commands more circulation to tap into its water content. The chemical messenger it uses to call for increased circulation is PGE-2 (prostaglandin-E 2). The more the pancreas has to rely on extra activity of PGE-2, the more it becomes critical that water not leave the circulation and enter the body cells as a companion to sugar and the amino acids. The resulting imbalance in the blood's water content is harmful to the brain, which has to maintain its 85 percent water content. This is why the brain cells do not possess insulin receptors and can pick up sugar and its water companion directly from the blood.

The natural design of pancreatic function is such that the more blood cannot deliver free water to the pancreas when PGE-2 calls for it, the more PGE-2 will inhibit insulin release by the beta-cells—thus the first stage of diabetes is produced in overweight

people. This kind of diabetes is labeled as type II or insulin-inde-
pendent diabetes, seen more among the elderly. In this form of diabetes, the pancreas contains lots of insulin, but does not release it.
This is when some chemicals that have been produced to overcome the action of PGE-2 can release some insulin to control the
blood sugar.

However, the body is better designed than we give it credit for. In
its next step to block the action of insulin, it covers the insulin
molecule with a substance called xanthurenic acid; this makes it
ineffective, because the insulin receptors will no longer recognize
it. This is when the tablet medications will no longer control blood
sugar levels and the use of insulin becomes unavoidable.

This is the simplified explanation of what John K suffered from—
and you saw how easily he reversed the problem. It naturally took
time to do so, but at least water made it possible.

Type I diabetes has a more drastic story, but is still a dehydration-
produced problem. It has to do with the process of remodeling and
cell cannibalism that the body resorts to when it is water- and
resource-depleted. Type I diabetics reduce their dependence on
insulin when they optimally hydrate their bodies. In this case, they
will also be saved from the drastic complications associated with
type I diabetes.

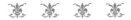

Note: The letter that follows is included here not for its story of
weight loss, but for all the other health miracles that water will
pass on to the person who drinks it regularly.

*I would like to thank you for your hard work in getting the information about
water out to the public. I have had such amazing results in just two weeks. I
was drinking four Cokes a day and maybe 16 to 32 ounces of water and lots
of chocolate. Everyone has been begging me to stop the Cokes but it didn't hit
home until I heard your program on the Art Bell show.*

I started on 80 ounces of water and 1/2 teaspoon salt the next day. I cut down to only two Cokes a day and I'm weaning off of them slowly because I'm so addicted. I was very nervous and irritated over the least thing that would happen. It seemed like I was headed for a nervous breakdown because of stress in my life. I couldn't sleep soundly and all of my joints were aching. Also, I felt my heart was very strained; whenever I would walk up steps or exert myself, I would be out of breath. I had sinus headaches and took two Sine-Aids every day, which I'm sure didn't help. My daughter just graduated from college and moved back home and I couldn't handle living with someone. My family and friends have been very concerned because I seemed to be losing self-control.

When I started the water and salt I couldn't believe the results. I feel laid back and calm like I used to be. I'm getting along great with my family and friends and they have commented on my changes and they have started the water also!! I have lost about five pounds without dieting and I feel a lot more energy. Not the spurts of energy I used to feel, but I'm not dead tired when I get off work at 11:45 PM. I have a little reserve tank left. But, when I am tired I can now sleep instead of feeling like my mind will not stop racing. I used to never feel thirsty, just wanted a lift. Now, I am thirsty and craving the water and have always had to force myself to drink water before. I will keep going and get off of the two Cokes and Sine-Aid and probably do even better. I ordered your tape on MS to pass on to three friends who have the disease. I will let you know what I hear back from them.

Sincerely, M. L.

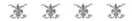

It is a pleasure to sit down and chronicle the effects that this lifestyle change has meant to me both professionally and personally.

On a professional basis, I was asked to listen to a tape called Your Body's Many Cries for Water. AWANE's executive director, Dick Healy, thought it important as manager of AWANE's Employee Assistance

Program to learn this health concept involving water. Dick also ordered additional books and videotapes for me to read and view.

The tape immediately created a desire for me to adopt its suggestions. I began this lifestyle change on June 10 and began drinking 2–3 gallons of water daily. Since that start date, I have

- *Lost 46 lbs.*
- *Blood pressure at normal—no meds needed*
- *Skin elasticity has returned*
- *Athlete's foot cured*
- *Asthma medication reduced*
- *Pain in lower back eliminated*
- *Foot pain eliminated*
- *Diabetes symptoms gone*

I have eliminated the diuretics mentioned in the book and have lost a taste or craving for those products.

I look forward to meeting you at our convention in December.

Yours truly, J. R.

Note: Taking 2 to 3 gallons of water a day is an exaggeration I do not recommend. Unless you know what you are doing, you might deplete the mineral reserves of your body. Stick to the recommendations that are made at the end of this book.

PART 2

DEPRESSION

CHAPTER 5

THE CHEMISTRY OF DEPRESSION

PERCEPTIVE MARKERS OF DEHYDRATION

When the body becomes dehydrated, the brain can still get water delivered by "raindrops" through the filter system in its cell membranes, but this is not enough to energize it as fully as when the body is hydrated. This discrepancy in the rate of water supply to the brain produces a certain number of sensory outcomes that I consider to be thirst perceptions. They are as follow:

THIRST PERCEPTIONS
- Feeling **Tired**
- Feeling **Flushed**
- Feeling **Irritable**
- Feeling **Anxious**
- Feeling **Dejected**
- Feeling **Depressed**
- Feeling **Inadequate**
- Feeling a **"Heavy Head"**
- **Cravings**
- **Agoraphobia**

Figure 5-1. This illustration should help you recognize the earlier stages of depression before it becomes deeply established. Bear in mind that untimely tiredness could be an early marker of depression. When you are too tired to get out of the bed first thing in the morning, you are in fact so dehydrated that your brain is refusing to get engaged in your daily routine. Water up and don't let the problem turn into full-blown depression.

WHAT IS DEPRESSION?

If it is the hot season and you are too preoccupied to water your grass, it will die of "brown grass disease." First the grass wilts; then patches of it begin to go yellow, and then brown. If these symptoms of dehydrated grass do not register in your mind the need to get out the water hose and thoroughly soak the yard, all the grass in your charge will die. And if, God forbid, the importance of water as a medication against the browning of grass and foliage is not held in the safekeeping of your brain, you might wonder what specialist could come and save you from having to re-grass your lawn. And, since specialists are by nature hard to come by and expensive, you would have no choice but to listen to their pearls of wisdom, particularly if the occurrence of brown grass disease is thought to be a genetic problem of the grass in your garden.

You would have no choice but to have the whole area of brown grass dug up and replanted with a different strain of grass. Since your new grass has to be watered to grow, you come away with the idea that your specialist knows what he's talking about, and totally in the dark that even your old grass needed to be watered regularly to stay green.

In its early stages, depression is like the brown grass disease of the brain cells. It is a direct outcome of not drinking water on a regular basis and, worse, of drinking caffeinated beverages in place of water. Caffeine is a drying agent and dehydrates the body. Nine trillion brain cells need water all the time. The brain is 85 percent water and needs every drop of it to perform its most complicated functions. Depression is much like the wilting stage of brown grass, but sadly, you cannot dig up the brain cells and plant new gene-improved models in their place, at least not yet. You will have to make do with what you have—water it.

Depression is only a label given to the physiological state of a dehydrated brain that is not able to perform all its sophisticated functions. Depending on what area of the brain is more affected by dehydration, different subsets of labels have generated for the same basic problem. And because jargon-peddling is the way of "knowledgeable professionals," the simple shortage of water, and the material resources it would bring with it for the needs of the brain, has been responsible for the creation of psychiatry as a field among the medical disciplines. The difference between psychology and psychiatry is in the way the patient is treated. In the one discipline they talk you out of your concerns, and in the other they medicate you into conformity.

Since you have been initiated into the field of psychiatry by the advertising programs of the drug industry, you likely want to know all about the relationship of water to serotonin and its reuptake inhibitors, and so on, before you can begin to value water as an effective natural medication against depression.

There are 20 amino acids. From these, the body manufactures different proteins for construction of both body tissues and the active messenger agents that regulate the body's functions. The body has the ability to manufacture 10 of these amino acids, but the other 10 cannot be manufactured and must be imported. The 10 amino acids the body can make are alanine, glycine, proline, serine, cysteine, aspartic acid, glutamic acid, asparagines, glutamine, and tyrosine. However, at least two of these amino acids—cysteine and tyrosine—are derivatives of other essential amino acids that the body cannot manufacture but must consume. Cysteine is manufactured from methionine, and tyrosine is manufactured from phenylalanine.

The body can manufacture some histidine, but not enough of it during childhood and old age. For this reason, histidine should also be considered an essential amino acid.

The essential amino acids—listed in the order of their importance for brain function—are histidine, tryptophan, phenylalanine, methionine, lysine, threonine, valine, arginine, leucine, and isoleucine.

Histidine gets converted to the neurotransmitter histamine and is responsible for the water regulation and resource management of the body. It operates your thirst sensations and regulates the water-rationing programs of the body. It is with us from minute one of life when the ovum is fertilized by the sperm, but has not yet divided into the two cells. Histamine has to "wet-nurse" the ovum for it to be able to expand in volume and then divide, and divide, until the baby is born—histamine is there all the time. In childhood, when the body is growing, histamine acts as a strong growth factor, much like growth hormone. The difference is that histamine becomes more and more active as we grow older, while growth hormone activity diminishes very rapidly from the third decade of life.

The tremendous need for the actions of histamine in childhood and old age makes its precursor amino acid, histidine, essential. Many neurological disorders, such as multiple sclerosis, seem to be produced because of histidine metabolism imbalance. Many emotional problems are associated with excess activity of histamine during its water-regulation.

The more the body becomes dehydrated, the more histamine activity takes over the physiological functions that were the responsibility of water. If there is not enough water to energize the mineral pumps, or cation pumps, and regulate the balance between sodium (which has to stay outside the cells) and potassium (which must be forced back in), histamine stimulates the release of energy to jump-start the protein pumps and bring about osmotic balance in the environment of the cells—most vitally in the brain.

Histamine acts as a natural energy manager in the absence of water and shortage of hydroelectric energy. Brain function is not efficient without histamine when the body is short of water. Nor is it efficient for long if it has to rely only on histamine as a substitute for the functions of water. In essence, this state of inefficient brain physiology, caused by the missing action of water, is what we call depression.

Histamine is in charge of the ionic balance inside the cells. It forces potassium ions that leak out of the cell wall back into the cell. It releases energy for the pumps that handles the process. The trigger mechanism that gets histamine going is a rise in the level of potassium in the environment around the cells, particularly the brain cells. In my opinion, the action of histamine in the body is what preserves life until water becomes available and can perform its natural functions: The use of antihistamine medications, when water itself is a better natural antihistamine, is tantamount to a criminal act. The tricyclic antidepressant medications, and in fact even the more modern antidepressants, function as very strong antihistamines.

The essential amino acid tryptophan gets converted into at least four neurotransmitters and hormones: serotonin, tryptamine, indolamine, and melatonin. Two enzymes, one unique to serotonin-producing cells and the other distributed more generally in the brain, act on tryptophan in this conversion process. Nature has selected tryptophan as the most important amino acid for the brain's control of all the sensations and functions of the body.

Serotonin is the kingpin chemical, needed for many events that silently regulate the body physiology. This is why a shortage of the serotonin that should normally be available is one of the hallmarks of depression. It's also why the pharmaceutical industry has produced a number of chemicals that slow down the rate of serotonin's destruction in the nerve terminals after it is secreted to perform one of its many functions:

- Serotonin alters the threshold of pain sensation and produces analgesia.
- Serotonin controls production and release of the growth hormone.
- Serotonin controls the level of blood sugar.
- Serotonin controls the blood pressure levels of the body—it

has a tendency to lower blood pressure.

- Serotonin and tryptophan control appetite. You remember I talked about motilin, which is considered a kind of gut serotonin. It is the hormone that causes the satiety sensation.

- Serotonin and tryptophan regulate the body's salt intake, whereas histamine controls the intake of potassium and its insertion into the cells.

- Serotonin has a direct effect on calcium movement into the cells and its involvement in neurotransmission.

- Serotonin release inhibits histamine's release and its action.

- Serotonin production by the brain is reduced when the blood levels of three amino acids—valine, leucine, and isoleucine—rise above normal, such as in starvation, dehydration, lack of exercise, and other conditions that affect protein metabolism of the body.

- Serotonin strengthens the contractile properties of certain muscles.

- The serotonin-stimulated nerve system (serotonergic system) is the medium through which analgesics such as morphine and hallucinogenic drugs like LSD register their effects. It is this kind of stimulation of the serotonergic system that becomes addictive when people get hooked on a drug, be it caffeine or cocaine.

The brain cells that convert tryptophan to serotonin have the ability to make this conversion at the same rate as it arrives. These cells do not store tryptophan itself, but store serotonin in vesicles and even pass these vesicles on the nerves' transport system down the track to the nerve endings, to be used when the nerve is stimulated. Thus, low serotonin levels in the nerve system—seen in depression—are only caused if tryptophan cannot be delivered to the nerve cells.

You now understand the physiological upheaval that occurs as a result of tryptophan shortage in the brain tissue. After 20-plus years of research into the relationship of water to pain regulation of the body, I have reached a broad understanding of how to avoid serotonin depletion in the brain and prevent depression.

WATER: NATURE'S ANTIDEPRESSANT MEDICATION

Directly or indirectly, water maintains an efficient and effective rate of tryptophan flow into the brain tissue for its immediate conversion into serotonin. Here's how:

- Normally, when the body gets dehydrated and cannot produce adequate urine to get rid of its toxic waste and the acid buildup in its cells, certain amino acids are sacrificed to neutralize this acid and make the body more alkaline. The term usually used is antioxidant. Tryptophan, tyrosine, cysteine, methionine, and more are all sacrificed in an attempt to keep the acid–alkali balance of the body chemistry within the normal range.

- Drinking enough water to create colorless urine—resulting in the washing of excess acid out of the body—would automatically conserve these essential amino acids, enabling them to perform their normal roles in the body. Thus adequate urine production, which should occur with water intake—not through the use of diuretics, caffeinated beverages, or alcoholic drinks—is a major safeguard against depression.

- All elements that need to get into the brain and reach its cells have to be carried on special transporter systems. These transporter systems are specific to various elements. Tryptophan shares its transporter system with five other amino acids: valine, leucine, isoleucine, phenylalanin, and tyrosine. The rate at which tryptophan can cross the blood–brain barrier (BBB) depends on the level of these other amino acids that are in circulation.

- In starvation, dehydration, and lack of exercise, blood levels of valine, leucine, and isoleucine increase. This reduces the available transport system for the passage of tryptophan across the BBB, thus causing a gradual depletion of the available tryptophan in the brain. If dehydration and lack of exercise become established trends in the lifestyle of any individual, the serotonin levels in the brain of that person will decrease.

- Valine, leucine, and isoleucine are energy-laden amino acids that can be used by the brain or the muscle tissues in the body for their energy needs—not to manufacture a product, but rather to perform a function. Exercise enables muscle tissue to mop up these amino acids from the circulation and make an intermediate product that the liver will then complete the process and make sugar for the brain to use. As a result of the muscles' collection of these amino acids from the circulating blood, increased space on transporter system (which exists only in the capillaries that feed the brain) is made available for the amino acid tryptophan to catch a ride and reach the brain side of the circulation.

- In the same way, the rate of tyrosine transfer to the brain side of the circulation will increase and cause a buildup of the dopamine levels that complement serotonin activity in the brain for increasing motivation and purpose. Thus, adequate exercise is an effective way to replenish brain serotonin levels and ward off depression.

- Another role of adequate hydration in boosting the serotonin levels of the brain is too complex to explain in this book. Briefly, tryptophan is extremely heat excitable. Water serves the purpose by producing high heat of activation at the cell membranes. This is most effectively done at the blood–brain barrier.

This local heat excites tryptophan. It dislodges itself from the transporter protein in the blood, and attaches itself to another transporter system in the wall of the better-hydrated brain capillaries. The new transporter system in the capillary wall will more efficiently and effectively deliver it to the brain. In the brain, it gets converted to serotonin, melatonin, tryptamine, and indolamine—the chemicals that regulate entire body physiology, including your mood and outlook on life.

With its simple local heat generation, water causes a speedier shift of tryptophan into the brain. Water also has many other indirect effects that help tryptophan reach into the brain cells. Thus, water is a natural medication against depression.

To prevent disease, you must prevent dehydration from getting established in the interior of your body's cells. To reverse a disease process, you need additional insight into the metabolic complications associated with prolonged water shortage in the body. Naturally, there are other treatment pointers that need to be followed. These are fully explained in the last three chapters of the book.

Having learned about the missing role of water in depression, let us now see some results.

STUPENDOUS RESULTS

I read your interview with Dr. Batmanghelidj a couple of weeks ago and it made a profound impression on me. I gave up beverages containing caffeine. Although I have only been on this program for a couple of weeks, I feel like a new person!

I wanted to tell you about some results that I got, because the ones that impressed me the most and for which I am most thankful, are not physical results, per se; they are emotional/psychological & mental.

I did get some very good physical results, I lost weight, my allergy symptoms disappeared, and I enjoyed a tremendous upsurge in energy—but I was much more grateful for (and amazed by) a release from a lifelong battle with depression, and other emotional and psychological problems. I had gotten to the point where my nerves were just shot. I was sensitive and overreacted to everything. The slightest setback became a major setback. I couldn't cope with the pressures of even ordinary everyday living, much less more stressful situations. I developed a very short fuse, I would get irritated and angry at the slightest provocation, and then I would get depressed and hated myself, and really just want to die. I was ruining my closest relationships, and I contemplated suicide many times. I began to believe that I might have a mental illness. I saw many different psychiatrists and social workers, but my experiences never really changed. I was progressively more volatile with drastic mood swings, and I lived under a big dark cloud. But then, when I began to follow Dr. Batmanghelidj's guidelines, I felt the big dark cloud lift. It was as if the sun finally came out. I felt calmer and more peaceful, more centered and grounded, and just plain happier.

My nerves no longer jumped out of control at every little thing and I began to feel a profound sense of joy and relief. I no longer felt so much like something was drastically wrong with me. I began to be able to hold my head up and face the world, instead of tending toward a sort of paranoid agoraphobia.

I don't know whether other people with similar problems might get the same relief, but as you say, when you've tried everything else and it's failed, it can't hurt to try something like this. I know many people who don't even drink one glass of water in a day. I can't imagine anyone who wouldn't benefit from increasing his or her intake of water.

Thank you so much for publishing that fascinating interview. It made more sense than anything else I have ever read on health (and I've read a lot), and it has helped me more than anything else I have ever tried (and I've tried a lot!).

Also, a glass of water is free—my last psychiatrist was $65.00 for 45 minutes!!

Thank you again,
Sincerely yours, K. M., Syracuse, New York

Note: As you can see, K. M. exhibited all the perceptive manifestations of dehydration that I identified in figure 5-1 at the beginning of this chapter. Once she corrected her daily intake of water to avoid dehydration, all those symptoms disappeared too.
I want to write and tell you of my health improvements since following

your water treatment. For the last 10 years I have suffered with chronic heartburn. I have been to many doctors, had numerous tests, even had my gallbladder removed and been prescribed several medications with no relief. I also have had a lifelong problem with depression, have tried many types of therapy and mind-altering drugs, and have been hospitalized. I have been seeing a homeopath, and he has helped me with several situations. He sent me a copy of your article in The Last Chance Health Report Vol. 3 #5, and suggested I also purchase your book Your Body's Many Cries for Water. He said he felt this would greatly help me. At that time, I had just been in the hospital having more tests, and was beginning a program of several strong medications. Some of which had dangerous potential side effects.

On August 24, 1993, I began drinking lots of water, 12 glasses on average and noticed dramatic improvement almost immediately. The heartburn was still occurring at the same rate, but I drank water and found it took 7 minutes for the heartburn to abate. I was dubious, to say the least, but decided not to take any medication and see what happened. After a week or so I noticed I had not been depressed either. This to me was amazing, considering all the advice I had been given in psychological counseling. A few days later, I realized I had not been having headaches as I usually did. I would have a slight headache on a daily basis. I've also noticed my skin is a lot clearer, I have more energy and overall I just feel better.

I have spent untold amounts of money, time away from work (I had used all my vacation time being sick) and energy dealing with medical doctors and hospitals, and receiving minimal relief. I am also in a few very stressful situations, but am able to cope. And I am taking no medication for heartburn or antidepressants. The episodes of heartburn are fewer now as well. The only change I've made is to drink lots of water. I have not yet begun the rest of your regimen, orange juice, etc., but intend to do so.

I feel like a different person, more in control of my life. It's now been two months and my skepticism is no longer there. I believe in your treatment. And want to thank you for it. I am now telling friends and co-workers to at least try it and have had good reports from them also. September 13, 1993, I had a follow-up appointment with my gastroenterologist, I told her I was feeling a lot better and gave her a copy of your article to read, she was nonplussed.

I am and have been very angry with the medical profession. Doctors for the most part do not even ask about your water intake or diet. Their methods ensure you a return appointment with lingering ailments and no education on being able to take care of yourself. Your treatment is simple, inexpensive, and it works! It is also a threat to medical doctors as they will see less of you and make less money. What I have been through is outrageous and insulting to my intelligence.

Thank you so much for enlightening me on how I can feel better without all the frustration, pain, and side effects I've experienced.

S. M.

✤   ✤   ✤   ✤

January 10, 2003

Dear Dr. Batmanghelidj,

Another friend this morning told me she just finished reading her copy of your wonderful book Your Body's Many Cries for Water, and shared the information with her young son who has bipolar and depression. He is drinking his water and also using light therapy and is no longer on any medication and feels wonderful. My daughter used to get legs cramps at night while sleeping but for the last three or four weeks has not had any cramping. I am feeling wonderful. No more wheezing and I sleep really well especially after I put a little salt on my tongue just before I fall asleep.

Sandra. Z

Dear Dr. Batmanghelidj:

Every day since I began your wonderful water & salt program, I read and reread your remarkable book Your Body's Many Cries for Water and continue to be impressed by the many ways in which your new paradigm brings to light the true etiology of the many diseases that are prevalent.

My excitement is mounting day by day, as I find my energy, clarity, and sense of well-being improving.

After struggling with debilitating chronic fatigue syndrome and acute depression for almost ten years now, I am very grateful for your remarkable insight and for your persistence in bringing this information to the public & scientific community.

I will be ordering a case of your paperbacks to send to friends and relations who are suffering from misdiagnosed illnesses.

May you live a very long life so that your research can continue and so that your teachings can spread around the world.

With deep appreciation,

D. G., Ph.D.

Subject: *My story: how many times do we need to hear the "stuff" before we get it. At the same time I am comforted knowing my Creator never gives up on me and the truth keeps returning!*

June 13 our car was rear-ended and both Jack and I were injured. Because I was turned (twisted so to speak) watching for oncoming traffic I received a whiplash to my hip. Did not feel hurt immediately, however 3 days later I felt like I had been beaten! Went to the chiropractor and massage therapist and acupuncturist . . . and with their treatments got periodic relief from the pain. Interestingly enough they would say, "drink water"; however, I made no connection with pain and dehydration! I have never taken so much Arnica even resorted to Advil some days, ice pack/heating pads . . . trochanteric belt, lumbar support belt . . . major depression.

What is going to happen! Then an article appeared 10 days ago in a local paper about Dr. B's work written by a local massage therapist and the connection of pain and dehydration . . . I thought I have nothing to lose. Next morning upon arising I immediately drank about 32 ounces of water and then continued throughout the day to get in about 80 ounces. About 3 days later I began to sense the pain diminishing. All this time I have been having treatments with some improvement but still the lingering pain.

After 5 days on the water I had an almost pain-free day! Then on the 6th day pain-free and have been since; truly it was the water, also lost a couple of pounds with no change to exercise or diet and my energy returned.

My depression lifted and I am back to my energetic loving self. So, yes, I am on a mission to spread the word and so glad you are doing such a fine job

Love Jeanne

Note: The letter that follows is about nine years old. The man who wrote it is well and is now using his knowledge of the WaterCure to advise older people in retirement homes. I am told he is very popular because he is making a difference in the lives of the people he meets.

Dear Dr. Batmanghelidj,

August 1995, I first became aware of your book Your Body's Many Cries for Water. I will be forever grateful for your years of research in reference to the role of water in the functioning of the human body. The chapter in the book pertaining to depression was the solution to over ten years of struggle in my life.

In your book, your simple formula of drinking water at the rate of minimum of two quarts (64 oz. = 8 glasses) per day plus salt of 1/2 teaspoon over a 24-hour period has been the answer for my depression. Because of my weight, I followed the additional suggested formula of half the body weight number = the ounces of water required to properly keep all the cells fully hydrated. I make sure that I ingest at least 1/2 a teaspoon of table salt (sodium chloride) with my food during the same 24-hour period.

I am a 68-year-old retired professional chemical engineer. I had battled depression symptoms from 1985 until 1995. My wife, a nurse clinician, passed away in 1984. I was forced into early retirement after 33 1/2 years with a major oil company in 1985. Those familiar with the role of high stress causing dehydration will understand my problem. In addition, I had bought into the idea that a low-salt diet was the way of good health. Thus, all the factors were in place for my body to show symptoms of depression.

What I now know is that most of the antidepressants used to treat patients with depression are also diuretics. I always manifested the symptom of extreme dry mouth sensation after being placed on antidepressants. The symptoms of anxiety then come forth because of the additional need for water by the body. Add a prescribed anti-anxiety pill and the patient (me) was on chemical teeter-totter trying to achieve a balance of a normal life. Plus, in the Physician's Desk Reference (PDR), in the listing for the above medications is the nice word, suicide. I have struggled when on antidepressants and anti-anxiety medication with the fleeting surges of the mind of wanting to die. However, I never had the courage to act out the desire. The ultimate solution, that worked for me: Water and salt; the simple answer.

In summary, for over a year I have been free of the need to take any medication of any kind. In December 1995, I qualified with no medical restrictions for a class physical for a private pilot's license. In addition, my annual eye check revealed that my peripheral vision had improved relative to previous annual tests. My belief is that the cells in my eyes have become better hydrated. I can now read without glasses.

May the value of your research and protocol continue to spread and to be understood.

Sincerely, Courtney Diddle, BS, Chemical Engineering

Note: I left Mr. Diddle's full name at the end of his letter because I am sure he would be delighted if people could benefit by his experience.

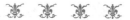

Dear Dr. Batmanghelidj,

I am writing to comment on and express my thanks for your research and your book Your Body's Many Cries for Water. I found it very concise and logical in its presentation and helpful in its message.

I would also like to relay my experience prior to reading your book and the implementation of drinking more water. I have no physical illness that I am aware of and enjoy good health, yet for all of my adult life I struggled with depressive states. These states are not predicable and I have found little effective remedy other than simply to endure and wait. Without describing my depression I can say that for me it was often near debilitating and I have as a consequence done considerable experimentation in an effort to find relief.

I have tried numerous therapies both additive and subtractive. In the additive, I've tried acupuncture, homeopathy, Chinese herbs, Western herbs, chiropractic, sound and color therapy, chemical drugs, vitamins, essential oils, more light, colon cleansing, ozone and oxygen supplements, meditation, individual and group psychotherapy, macrobiotic diet, and more exercise. In the subtraction I have eliminated amalgam fillings, caffeine, meat and sugar, alcohol and drugs, and all foods, during certain periods in my life.

In regard to the effects of these trials I can say that only the increasing exposure to natural sunlight and use of antidepressant chemical drugs have had a noticeable effect on my depression. I still get more sunlight but have abandoned drugs due to unacceptable side effects and concerns over long-term dependency.

I read Cries for Water nearly three months ago and started drinking at least 8 glasses of water a day two months ago. I think that after this time I can with relative certainty say that there has been a marked improvement in my mood and absence of depressive states. This I say as a general statement. There are times when I feel low but on the whole I feel much improved. I have much humor and my thoughts are much more optimistic. I have observed that even a single day without drinking water has a negative effect.

I feel compelled to thank you for your work and for bringing it to the public. Although I cannot comment on the relationship between drinking more water and other maladies I would not hesitate to recommend the book and the practice of drinking more water to anyone who struggles with depression.

Cordially, J. W.

Note: I downloaded the next testimonial from the review section of an Internet site. It was so poignant that I could not resist sharing it with you. I hope the author does not mind. I am sure he would want you to read it, too.

Don't listen to the negative reviews—try it yourself!

March 5, 2004
Reviewer: aggressivepeace from San Francisco, CA

I think Mr. Urologist (I won't use Dr.) has no clue what he is talking about. I have no medical degree and can tell you that what he is saying is asinine. Water intoxication, in most cases, is found in triathletes, marathoners, and military. It only happens when they have drunk excessive (generally over 200 ounces) amounts in a small period of time. This caused their sodium and mineral balances to go awry and they got sick or died. If the Pee Doctor had actually read the book, he would see that Dr. Batman talks repeatedly about adding sea salt to your intake if you have concerns about water intoxication.

I have had the following benefits from increasing my water intake to half my body weight in ounces per day, plus an additional 1.5 ounces of water for every 1 ounce of caffeinated beverages. (For me this is 128 ounces of water a day, I weigh 220 and drink one 12-ounce soda a day.) Again, follows is a list of the benefits I have had, if you don't believe me you are foolish. I have no reason to lie.

- *no depression*
- *more energy*
- *sleeping better*
- *skin more elastic and generally healthier (I am getting compliments about my face)*
- *increased sense of well-being or doing something positive for myself*
- *full, clear urine*

- *full, regular excrement*
- *no back pain (lower)*
- *reduced knee/joint pain*
- *less pain in my damaged ulnar nerve*
- *eat less*
- *feel tired less*
- *awareness of thirst has returned (I don't eat or do something else instead)*
- *less heartburn*

The absolute most positive and main effect is no depression. I am entirely astounded at the positive effect this has had on my life. I have gotten off meds and will never return, for now I know the true answer. Meds are good to get you through a bad spot, but they will not relieve your depression effectively over a long period of time. This doesn't even consider the horrible side effects.

It is so clear that this is the healthiest thing that you can ever do for yourself (a close #2 is regular cardiovascular and muscle-building exercise). I personally commit that you will have increased health and mentality if you drink the correct amount of water for yourself. Also, consult Dr. Weil regarding the power of your mind toward your health.

Peace and good hydration to you all.

Thanks Dr. Batman!!!!!! You are a life saver. I hope your message gets to more and more people. I am now having friends come back to me stating how they are noticing differences for themselves. No one really believes it until it happens to them, and when my friends saw the sincerity I had about my improvement they tried it themselves.

Thanks again. You have truly made the world a better place.

The next letter is from someone who is daily seeing sick people and curing them with water. His story is interesting.

The Center for Functional Nutrition
514 Amherst Road, South Hadley, MA 01075
413-536-0275
www.healthequest.com
maramor1@earthlink.net
Russell Mariani, M.A., Director of Client Education Services

F. Batmanghelidj, M.D.

September 21, 2004

Dear Dr. B,

This is a letter that is long overdue!

Since 1973, when I was incorrectly diagnosed with colon cancer and then ineffectively treated for ulcerative colitis, I have been on a quest to discover the fundamental connections between our nutritional choices and our health. Scientific studies, though often helpful, should never be a replacement for our own direct personal experiences. Thank you for encouraging people to take more responsibility for our own health and well-being by taking actions that truly nourish us best.

In my own experience, I was shocked to discover how little I understood about the cause and effect relationships between states of chronic unintentional dehydration and disease. Even in my natural healing classes I had been advised to eat when you're hungry and drink when you're thirsty. I had been taught that there was enough water content in the cooked whole grains, steamed vegetables and fresh fruits that I was eating and that extra water was rarely necessary. I was taught that drinking water would dilute and render ineffective the digestive juices. I was taught that drinking water would weaken the kidneys. How incorrect all that advice turned out to be! Although I had always made a point of drinking only fresh spring-water or purified tap water, there were many years of my life that I rarely drank more than one or two glasses of water per day. For most of the past thirty years, I have weighed an average of two hundred pounds. So you can see that my daily water intake had been woefully inadequate for a very long time.

My body was constantly crying out to me for water and salt, but I did not know how to interpret these messages. Irritable bowel, chronic fatigue, dry skin, days of acute anxiety, weeks of constant depression, periodic kidney stones; were all signals of thirst and chronic dehydration that I missed for many, many years. More importantly, because of my own ignorance of the role of proper daily hydration and health, I was unable to pass this vital information on to others. Fortunately, all of that changed about seven years ago.

In the middle of one of the worst episodes of acute anxiety and constant depression in my life, someone handed me your first book: Your Body's Many Cries for Water. After reading chapter 5 on Stress and Depression, I had the thought: "Why haven't I ever read or heard anything about this before?" Your explanations all made perfect sense. A few days later I phoned your office and spoke to you in person. You simply advised me to begin measuring the inflow of water and the outflow of urine, and to consume half my body weight in ounces of water with salt, daily. Thus began one of the most helpful and important learning experiences of my life.

Following your sage advice, it took a mere twenty-one days for my body to rid itself of the state of anxiety and depression that I had been suffering from for almost two months.

Remember, that I had been suffering from periodic (and medically unexplainable) bouts of anxiety and depression for over twenty years. In the previous three years, I had also started to experience the excruciating pain of kidney stones, which came upon me like clockwork in the late summers of 1994, 1995 and 1996.

Since first learning about the WaterCure in March, 1997, I have not had one relapse of anxiety or depression. I have not had another kidney stone attack either. I know with absolute confidence and certainty that both of these medically unexplainable conditions had their origin in my state of chronic unintentional dehydration. As the weeks and months and years roll by, the benefits of proper daily hydration continue to manifest.

Clearly there exists no more powerful medicine on earth than simple water and salt! Clearly, the easiest thing each one of us can do every single day to ensure the highest quality of health inside our own bodies, is to maintain proper hydration levels within the cells, organs and systems, by drinking the correct amounts of water with salt. In the hierarchy of effective health solutions, nothing is more important than water with salt. The WaterCure is health solution number one!

I have tried many natural, alternative and holistic health habits for over thirty years now, and all of them have worked to one degree or another. Water with salt is the thing that ties them all together. When the body is properly hydrated on a daily basis, every other complementary health practice is enhanced and made more effective. For many people this habit of water with salt is the missing piece of the puzzle in their long search for effective health solutions. In my work with clients in my nutrition counseling practice, it is the very first thing I teach them. Please let your readers know that they are welcome to contact me by phone or e-mail at any time. I am committed to helping you get the word out about proper daily hydration. The WaterCure is not only vital; it's transformational.

Thank you for your pioneering work in educating the world about the role of proper daily hydration and health. Ignorance truly is the cause of all human suffering. And education, of the kind you continue to provide us all, is the very best medicine we have.

Sincerely, Russell Mariani

PART 3

CANCER

CHAPTER 6

WHY ME?

When I discovered in 1980 that water has pain-relieving properties, even when the afflicted reach a semiconscious state of mind—what I have called pain stupor—it became clear to me that water was an enigma to us in the medical profession and needed to be studied. After 24 years of full-time research into the molecular physiology of dehydration—a topic of research developed and published by me—I still think water is an enigma that needs our focused attention in medical research. However, my findings about water so far are sufficiently mature and well reviewed that I feel safe in sharing them with scientists and the lay public. Here are some of the highlights of my findings about the relationship between dehydration and cancer formation in the body.

I first presented these findings as the guest lecturer at an international cancer conference in 1987 in Greece, and published them in the *Journal of Anticancer Research* in October 1987 (Pain: A Need for Paradigm Change; *Anticancer Research* 7, no. 5B, Sept.–Oct. 1987, 971–990; full article posted on www.watercure.com).

My new perspective on pain as an indicator of dehydration attracted the attention of some serious scientists in Europe. I was invited by the Scientific Secretariat of "The 3rd Interscience World Conference on Inflammation and Immune Modulators" to present my newly highlighted understanding of histamine as the primary neurotransmitter in charge of water regulation and the drought-management programs of the body. I was asked to address the attending scientists in the main auditorium of the conference in March 1989 in Monte Carlo. Below is the abstract of my presenta-

3rd INTERSCIENCE WORLD CONFERENCE ON
INFLAMMATION
ANTIRHEUMATICS, ANALGESICS,
IMMUNOMODULATORS.

ABSTRACT FORM

IMPORTANT: These instructions must be followed completely.
Read all instructions before you begin typing on this special
form.

Mail to
Scientific Secretariat
3rd Interscience
World Conference
on Inflammation
Istituto di Farmacologia
Via Roma, 55
56100 Pisa (Italy)

Published JANUARY 30, 1989
Deadline: JANUARY 30, 1989

Title

NEUROTRANSMITTER HISTAMINE :
AN ALTERNATIVE VIEW POINT

Authors

F. Batmanghelidj, M.D.

Foundation For The Simple In Medicine,

2146 Kings Garden Way, Falls Church, VA. 22043, U.S.A.

Institute

ABSTRACT: Advances in histamine research show it to be a neurotransmitter, a neuromodulator and an osmoregulator of the body. While thirst sensation is a failing indicator of now recognized, age-dependent, state of possible cellular and chronic dehydration of the body, to the point that between the ages of twenty to seventy the ratio of the extracellular to the intracellular water content of the body has been shown to change from a figure of 0.8 to almost 1.1, histamine is demonstrating responsibility for the essential osmoregulatory and central dipsogenic functions in the body. Histamine is involved in the initiation of cellular cation exchange, that seems to be supplemental to the role of water in cellular metabolic mechanisms. Histamine is also a modulator of lymphocyte biology and function; through H_1 or H_2 activation of the different lymphocyte subpopulations that have nonrandom distribution of histamine receptors, their functions are integrated. Histaminergic drive for body water regulation and intake brings about the release of vasopressin, which in turn, by possible production of "shower head" cluster perforations of 2 Angstrom units, allowing single file entry of one water molecule at a time through the membrane, promotes increased flow of water through the cell membrane; this function is particularly important for the maintenance of the low viscosity, microtubule directed, microstream flow of the axonal transport system. Vasopressin seem also to act as a modulating cortisone release factor, when constant ACTH secretion can be implicated in the general inhibition of the immune system's functions; histamine may be involved in modulation of neuroendocrine systems, possibly when ACTH feedback mechanism is broken. Next to oxygen water is the single most essential substance for the survival of the body, also recognizing that the dry mouth is not the sole indicator of "free water" deficiency of the body, symptom producing excess histaminergic activity, including chronic pain production, should be judged to be also an indicator of body water metabolism imbalance. The natural primary physiological drives of the histaminergic, the serotonergic neurotransmission (another system involved in the body water regulation, as well as pain threshold alteration) and the angiotensin II for water intake of the body should be acknowledged and satisfied before and during evaluation of the clinical application of antihistamines in treatment procedures, particularly as increased water intake may be the only natural process for the regulation and inhibition of histamine's over production and release. The prolonged use of antihistamines in gastroenterological, psychiatric, seasonal allergic conditions, as analgesics or anti-inflammatory agents without very strict attention to body water intake regulatory functions of histamine, by also masking signals of dehydration, may eventually be the cause of cell membrane receptor down-regulation and disturb the integration and balance, and possibly, shift the immune system in an opposite dominant direction and therefore, be responsible for the production of new and continuing change of physiological steady-state situations, incompatible with the total and prolonged well-being of the patient.

Key Words: *Histamine, pain, inflammation, immunomodulation, thirst, water*

FORMAT FOR ABSTRACT

1. Your abstract should be informative, containing: (a) specific objectives; (b) methods; (c) summary of results; (d) conclusions.
2. Single space all typing. Capitalize all letters of the title. The text should be a single paragraph, starting with a 3-space indentation. Leave no top or left margin within the area provided.
3. Abbreviations must be spelled out on first mention, followed by the abbreviation in parentheses.
4. Any special symbol that is not on your typewriter must be drawn in BLACK INK.
5. DO NOT ERASE. Remember that your abstract will appear in a special volume exactly as submitted.
6. Mail first class with 2 photocopies to address given above.
7. If more than one abstract is submitted with the same first author, indicate which abstract should have priority. Other abstracts will have a lower priority.
8. **Please underline speaker's name.**

PUBLISHED; PAGE 37 OF THE ABSTRACT VOL.
3rd Interscience World Conference On Inflammation,
Antirheumatics, Analgesics,Immunomodulators.
Monte-Carlo (Principality Of Monaco), March 15-18, 1989
In Win 89

tion, which was published in their book of abstracts.

As you see, I am recognized for my development of a new scientific understanding of chronic unintentional dehydration as the primary cause of pain and disease, including cancer formation in the human body.

In the interim, these findings were further developed and consolidated by the work we did in the Foundation for the Simple in Medicine. We published our findings in the Journal of Science in Medicine Simplified—the same journal that the National Library of Medicine refused to index because their NIH panel member asked them not to.

In the meantime, the information on dehydration and cancer underwent serendipitous independent testing by the time it was presented at the 2002 Cancer Control Society conference in Los Angeles. A videotape of this presentation—Dehydration and Cancer—is available at www.watercure.com.

There is a direct relationship between dehydration—what I perceive as lasting, deep dehydration in the interior of the cells, not the traditionally understood dehydration from the environment around the body cells—and nearly 100 major and minor health problems in the human body. You've already read that obesity and depression are complications of dehydration. In this section, I will try to explain, in simple terms, why cancer is also the outcome of water shortage. To pique your interest and to show that the WaterCure works for cancer, let me begin by sharing with you an e-mail I received from Patrick M. on how his prostate biopsy was cancer-free even when his PSA was high.

"I want to thank you—I just got the biopsy result from the biopsy done on my prostate and they showed "absolutely no sign of cancer." My doctor had warned me that my PSA (prostate blood test) was very high and the "free factor" very low—an indication I had cancer. I had been on the WaterCure program and so was disappointed. I know now that the program is valid and thank you for your support. I will get even more serious and never give up drinking my 100 oz a day. Regards Patrick

Let us now see why water is a preventive medication against cancer.

WHAT IS CANCER, AND
WHY DOES IT EVENTUALLY KILL?

Cancer is a "selfish," invasive type of tissue that develops within an organ of the body. It breaks the natural boundaries of the mother organ and eventually spreads rapidly, disproportionately, and invasively, resulting in fatal disruption of normal body functions, to the point of exhaustion and death. What is the difference between cancer cells and other ordinary cells in the same organ?

Cancer Cells

1 - Primitive & Genetically Selfish
2- Anaerobic — Low Oxygen Needs
3- Reveal Stem Cell
Characteristics in some
Cell Culture Media.

Figure 6-1. The natural characteristics of cancer cells.

As the cells in the body mature, they develop sophisticated communication skills. They develop all kinds of receivers and sensors on their membranes. These sensors are needed to coordinate the cell's activity with the rest of the body. They integrate the cell and its specialized activity into the larger scheme of body physiology. One class of sensors on the cell membrane controls the boundaries up to which the cell will grow and not beyond. These sensors feel the presence of the other cells in their proximity. They maintain a safe distance from neighboring cells via the messaging system between the membrane receptors and the DNA mechanisms of the cell that control its growth and reproduction.

In this mode of their "socially sophisticated" life, the cells of the body are normally respectful of the other cells and are not "selfish."

They do not encroach on the rights of the other cells in their vicinity. Cancer cells have lost these social skills, however. Such cells grow into a mass that breaks boundaries and encroaches on the space normally allocated to neighboring tissues. The process in which the efficiency of these sensors is reduced and eventually lost, to the point of forming cancerous growths, is called receptor down-regulation. I will later explain why this kind of receptor loss from the cell membrane is another complication of unintentional dehydration.

Cancer cells are anaerobic and can only live in low-oxygen and acidic environments—the exact outcomes of low water flow and inefficient environmental cleanup. The acid by-products of metabolism are not washed away efficiently and regularly because of inefficient microcirculation in the region of cancer cells. The water flow of the blood should also bring oxygen to the area. Thus, the consequential environmental change, when the cleansing process is inefficient, predisposes the conversion of normal cells in the affected area to new cell types that thrive in an otherwise hostile and insufficiently oxygenated local environment.

Cancer cells have stem cell characteristics. They have the capability to achieve sophistication and develop specialized characteristics of normal cells.

Thus, the loss of cell membrane sensors and the conversion of sophisticated cells into primitive and selfish cells that thrive in a low-oxygen and acidic medium is the first step to cancer formation. For these transformed cells to develop into a cancer cell mass, however, three other major control mechanisms must also be disrupted. In other words, cancer formation in the body is the product of a multisystem physiological disruption. I will now explain why chronic unintentional dehydration is at the root of the entire problem.

Cancer-Controlling Systems of the Body

Dehydration-produced physiological factors predisposed to cancer cell formation

A multifactorial system dysfunction

- **DNA damage**

- **Reduced efficiency of DNA repair system**

- **Receptor down regulation and receptor up regulation**

- **Immune system supression**

Figure 6-2. Important cancer-preventing systems that do
not function normally when the body is not
optimally hydrated.

There is more to cancer formation and growth than one item; one
particle; one carcinogen; one external factor, such as sunlight; or
any one thing, except lack of sufficient water intake and its secondary complications. Cancer is truly the product of a drastic disruption in several major control mechanisms in the body. If only
one of them were in place, cancer cells would not be able to sur-

vive and thrive.

DNA DAMAGE:
A PREREQUISITE TO CANCER FORMATION

The human body is a satellite of water-dependent units of life—about 100 trillion of them housed together in one capsule on their journey of life on land. The cells of the body, each endowed with the same genetic secrets of life, have accepted a division of labor for an orderly conduct of business in their collective land-based shelter—the body. It has an intricate water-dependent design—a mobile water-regulated chemical refinery that has established a foothold on dry land. Medical pundits have misunderstood the various ways the body deals with its inner cleansing processes. But nonetheless, they pontificate commerce-suited solutions to different pain sensations, without the slightest understanding of why the body, at times, manifests such diverse localized or general pains.

The new science of medicine has identified pain as a signal of water shortage in the vicinity of where pain is felt—the crisis thirst signals of the body. Just as a drought threatens the survival of the local vegetation, a drought in the interior of the body threatens the survival of life in the drought-stricken areas of the body. Symbolically, pain is the cry of the gene pool in the drought-stricken area that cannot be washed and cleansed from destructive local toxic waste. Fortunately, the body possesses a strict water-rationing program that delivers some water to preserve life, but not enough for the other toxic waste-producing functions that would cause further pain. This is the reason pain limits function until more water comes on board and can be distributed to offset the local drought.

The mechanism of pain production is a simple process. When there is not enough water circulation to cleanse the toxic waste of continuous function from the drought-stricken area and acid by-products of metabolism continue to build up, at a certain level of acidity—a level that obviously eats into and hurts the gene pool—an acid-sensitive substance in the nerve tissue called kininogen gets converted to kinin. Kinin itself is a pain-producing substance.

The pain sensors and nerve endings in the area register their toxicity information with the brain, and the brain translates this message for the conscious mind into attention-grabbing pain. It next stops further activity in the area of pain until the circulation opens up and more blood is brought to cleanse the area and activate the repair processes to undo the damage. This process causes a localized inflammatory reaction, be it in the joints of the hands and the legs, the spinal column, the heart muscle (angina), and all the other pains listed below.

Many of the major pains of the body denote localized thirst. Heartburn in the upper parts of the intestinal tract, and colitis pain and its companion constipation in the lower intestinal tract—which predispose to cancers of stomach, esophagus, colon, rectum, and their pancreatic water-distributing organ—are the most frequently seen thirst pains of the body. The pancreas is responsible for giving priority to the intestinal tract for its water-distribution mechanisms. Primarily, it manufactures a watery bicarbonate solution and injects it into the first part of the small intestine. Not only does this alkaline, enzyme-laden watery solution neutralize the acid from the stomach, but it also constantly irrigates the intestinal walls during the digestive process. As it was explained, its rate of insulin production is dependent on the amount of water that reaches the pancreas.

When the body gets more and more dehydrated, insulin release is reduced until full-blown diabetes develops. With unintegrated insulin release and without considering the body's state of hydration, much water also leaves the blood along with the sugar that enters all cells of the body through their insulin receptor openings. Such an uncontrolled loss of water from circulation, in a dehydrated state, limits the amount of water that reaches the brain, and that is a no-no for the integrity of brain function.

As far as I understand, during the immediately prediabetic phase of function, or its post-diabetic phase of insulin shutdown, pancreatic cancers are also associated with dehydration. I am of the opinion that type I diabetes—the kind you must inject insulin to control, even though it is classified as an autoimmune disease—is another of the many complications of dehydration. Autoimmune diseases are also dehydration produced. It seems dehydration-produced cancers are more frequent in tissues that have secretory functions, like the intestinal tract, the breast, or the pancreas.

Other pains are also related to dehydration:

- Arthritis pain of the hand, arm, and leg joints.
- Back and neck pain.
- Migraine headaches. These should be taken as a serious indicator of "brain thirst" that herald eventual disruption of brain function, including brain tumors or degenerative diseases such as MS, Parkinson's disease, and even Alzheimer's disease.
- Angina.
- Fibromyalgia, denoting acid buildup in the muscles and the connective tissue—the locomotive faculties of the body.
- And more.

Adequate rehydration should be the first step toward pain relief. Hydration is a godsend solution for these pains. Take it from me and test water as a natural painkiller.

It has become an established trend to silence the pains of the body with some sort of chemical without knowing the wider physiological implications of the pain mechanism and its significant association with the level of acidity in the body. Pain means that an area is acidic. This can cause severe damage to the DNA structure of the cells within the area.

Medical specialists limit their responsibility to one aspect or another of the body's mechanical parts, and do not simultaneously deal with different diseases. They have mostly forgotten their knowledge of physiology and have acquired the skills of producing temporary relief by the use of chemical products. However, when pain medications are used, the cause of pain is not taken away; the acidic state of the body continues to cause other symptoms and damage that may be outside a specialist's field of interest. Thus patients go from one specialist to another and end up using several different chemicals to deal with their body's increasing variety of cries for water. Cancer formation is one such cry for water. It is the survival strategy installed in the primitive form of single-cell life in a chemically hostile environment.

It's true that many people develop cancer without having had pain. How can this be? Pain is one of many indicators of dehydration in the body. Not all parts of the body that become dehydrated possess pain-sensing nerves—think of the breast, the pancreas, the prostate gland, the lungs—hence their silent cancers. Water distribution is a highly sophisticated process operated on the basis of a very strict rationing program. The level of dehydration might be subclinical—without symptoms—but sufficiently present over a period of many years to cause damage to the DNA repair system, decrease the rate of receptor production on the cell membranes, and eventually negatively affect the immune system's efficiency of functions.

The onset of dehydration might well be established with the first prescription of diuretics to lower the blood pressure, without the doctor realizing that hypertension itself is one of the indicators of dehydration—one of the body's drought-management programs. Water has to be forced into vital cells against the osmotic draw of blood pulling water out of them; extra pressure is needed to inject some water through "water-specific holes" in the membranes of these vital but dehydrated cells.

In short, the rise in injection pressure of the emergency water distribution system in a dehydrated body is labeled hypertension. It is treated with chemicals that further dehydrate—diuretics—when water itself is the best natural diuretic there is. Can you imagine that? Yes! In this most advanced country in the world, more than 60 million dehydrated people have been labeled as hypertensives and receive this kind of treatment every day. No wonder heart disease and cancer are the number one and two killers—over 700,000 thousand die of heart disease and more than 500,000 die of cancer each year. Not surprisingly, over 250,000 die of prescription medications.

REDUCED EFFICIENCY OF DNA REPAIR SYSTEMS

Normally, the kidneys regulate the balance between acid and alkaline states of the body fluids, provided they receive enough water to produce a good amount of urine. The pH in the interior of the cells is regulated at 7.4—an alkaline state. When the body becomes more and more dehydrated and urine production is diminished, the mechanism of acid–alkaline balance becomes inefficient. The acid is not collected from some of the areas outside the emergency water distribution programs; it stays in the cells and eats into their delicate structures. This is when DNA damage takes place, repeatedly and often. Eventually, but surely, the destructive rate of excessive acidity outstrips the ability of the DNA repair systems and the quality-control processes installed in the cells. This is when DNA transformation takes place.

At the same time, when the body becomes dehydrated and insufficient raw materials are made available to vital cells, the body has to release some of its stored elements and use them on an emergency basis in whatever capacity they can function. As part of this process, proteins are broken down and their amino acids are recycled and used in new capacities.

A number of these amino acids act as antioxidants and neutralize the acidic toxic waste that has built up in the body. Among the amino acids that may gradually become depleted, because they are sacrificed as antioxidants, tryptophan is perhaps most precious. Tyrosine—the building block for a number of "go-getter" neurotransmitters—is another amino acid that gets abused when the body is short of water.

Tryptophan converts in the brain and the nervous system to serotonin, melatonin, tryptamine, and indolamine, all vital neurotransmitters. Low serotonin levels are associated with severe depression. Tryptophan is also coupled with two lysines—another amino acid that gets easily destroyed when the body is dehydrated—to form a tripod enzyme that has an intricate role within the quality-control system of the DNA transcription process (see figure 6-3). This enzyme is said to engage in cutting and splicing transcription errors in newly forming cells.

Thus, a dehydration-induced run on the tryptophan reserves of the body can result initially in depression and contribute to eventual cancer cell production in some parts of the body. Serotonin also regulates blood pressure, blood sugar levels, salt balance, and growth hormone production. You can now see the devastating effect dehydration has on the normal functions of the body, and how so many health problems are related events.

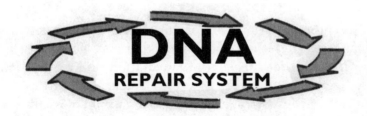

DEHYDRATION ALSO PROMOTES
PROTEIN BREAKDOWN

AMINO ACID COMPOSITION IS AFFECTED

TRYPTOPHAN, TYROSINE AND OTHERS
MAY BECOME DEPLETED

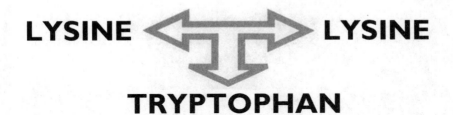

LYSINE   **LYSINE**

TRYPTOPHAN

**THE TRIPOD SYSTEM FOR DNA QUALITY
CONTROL AND REPAIR**

Figure 6-3. The vitally important role of tryptophan in the DNA
repair system that is affected by unintentional dehydration.

RECEPTOR DOWN-REGULATION

What are receptors and what relationship do they have to dehydration and cancers? These are the questions that need answers before
we can buy into the idea that simple dehydration could, over a fairly extended period of time, predispose to cancer. The process is a
gradual erosion of the controlling systems that would normally prevent ongoing deviations from the norms of the body.

We use receiver dishes for electronic communication through the
air. Working on a similar principle, the human body uses special
kinds of receiver proteins on the membranes of its nearly 100 trillion
cells in their watery environment. They constantly receive specially
coded chemical messages that get attracted to their messenger-specific receptors in their fluid environment. The purpose of the union
of the messenger chemical with its receptor on the cell membrane is
code-specific communication with the command centers in the
brain. The message system is simple. It tells some groups of cells to
act, or stop activity; hence the reason for possessing so many different chemical messengers for different subsets of cells (see figure 6-4).
The presence of adequate messenger-specific receptors on the membranes of a cell is a prerequisite to its normal operation.

A healthy cell is well endowed with protein receptors on its membranes. The health of any cell depends on its rate of protein production as compared with its recycling process of protein breakdown.
There are two kinds of protein-specific enzymes. The protein kinase
group of enzymes engages in protein manufacture, and the protease
group engages in the breakdown of proteins. In dehydration, the
resource-management programs begin to recycle some of the protein reserves of the body. To do so, protease activity and the rate of

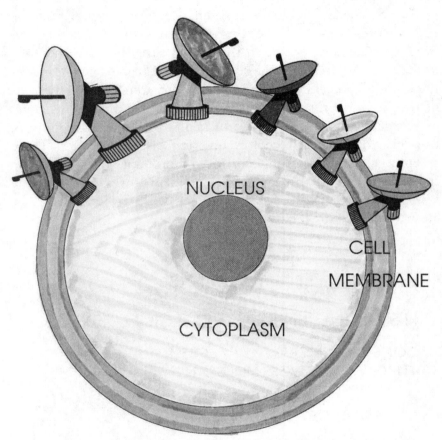

NUCLEUS

CELL

MEMBRANE

CYTOPLASM

EACH CELL HAS MILLIONS OF
RECEPTOR LIKE SATELLITE DISHES

Figure 6-4. Normal cells possess receptors on their membranes
that receive information from the rest of the body.

protein breakdown will overtake the rate of protein production. The way this is done is simple. When histamine breaks into the energy reserves in the calcium deposits in the cells—and eventually in the bones—to release needed extra energy, much loose calcium is produced. The excess calcium release is a signal that the energy stores of the body are getting depleted, and that other energy-containing components in the protein structures—such as the muscle tissue—are also being used. The proteases become mobilized, initially breaking into the protein structures within the cells of the water-deprived areas and the liver; eventually the larger muscle mass in the body gets attacked. The protein structures of the cells include the receptors on their cell membranes. These receptors include the boundary-sensing proteins that would stop the cell growth into the neighboring cell's physical space. With the loss of such sensors, the potential tumor cells grow disproportionately into large, irregular lumps.

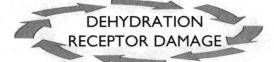

DEHYDRATION
RECEPTOR DAMAGE

HISTAMINE INCREASES CALCIUM RELEASE

CONSTANT INCREASED CALCIUM
TUROVER INCREASES MEMBRANE
PROTEASES

RECEPTORS DESTROYED

PROTEIN KINASE **C** BROKEN TO
PROTEIN KINASE **M**

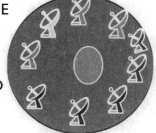

IRREGULAR PROTEIN PRODUCTION

CELL BECOMES AUTONOMOUS

Figure 6-5. Enzymatic changes destroy the receptors that should
normally be represented on a cell membrane to receive
communications from the rest of the body. The cell is
now isolated—the first step toward cancer formation.

At the beginning, this kind of growth may not necessarily be cancerous and may still remain benign; still, the tendency for the benign tumor to transform into full-blown cancer is there, if physiological events continue to progress in that direction. This will happen when the next stage of protein breakdown inside the cell and within the DNA transcription system takes place.

Protein kinase-C is a largish-sized protein-making enzyme connected to the DNA transcription process. It is found in normally active cells. It is responsive to the on–off switching processes within the cell—it is integrated in the physiological roles of the cell in its residing organ. Naturally, this kinase is efficient when the primary amino acids it works with are sufficiently available in the body and adequately present in the cell. It uses these amino acids for the manufacture of essential components of the cell, such as its membrane receptors.

The membrane receptors bestow "personality," "culture," and "knowledge" on the cell. Cells that are endowed with a full array of receptors are educated and sophisticated cells. Such cells are members of the team of cells that respond to the needs of the organ—finely tuned into their roles.

When the proteases begin to break down the receptor components of the cell, they also break down protein kinase-C and ultimately create a new kinase—protein kinase-M. Protein kinase-M is half the size of protein kinase-C and is totally disobedient to the on–off calls of the cell. It is an autonomous protein-making enzyme that gets gradually phased into the daily life of the cell.

This is when the cell regresses into its earlier, primitive form of itself, losing its sophistication and its status as an integrated member of the local cell community. It is now only obedient to its selfish genetic drive to survive at any cost. Much like the primitive single stem cell life-form at the start of life—a breed of genetically selfish cells with a powerful will to survive in their hostile, low-oxygen, concentrated, and acidic physiological environment. Later these cells acquired sophistication and secondary characteristics compatible with their environmental change.

It might just be possible for the cancer cells to also achieve their previous sophistication and secondary characteristics if the local conditions and availability of raw materials revert to normal. They might once again regain their sophistication with optimization of their environmental conditions. After all, they have all the genetic apparatus to do so. I believe that this is exactly what happens when cancers go into remission.

Cancer cells demonstrate stem cell characteristics in cell cultures. Stem cells are the "mother cells" that give rise to new breeds of cells, which are then sent to new environments to mature. In their new environment, they develop secondary characteristics and are then distributed for their ultimate working instructions.

Let me give you an example. Please bear with me, because understanding this process will help you see how lymphomas and leukemia are also associated with dehydration.

As you know, histamine is a neurotransmitter that regulates water intake and its rationing programs when the body is dehydrated. There are four kinds of histamine-producing cells—histamine-producing neurons in the brain, basophil lymphocytes in blood, mucosal mast cells in the intestinal tract, and tissue mast cells in the other organs of the body. Bone marrow stem cells give off a branch that is destined to become histamine-producing cells. Before they go through their schooling process, they are called P-cells. P-cells are a kind of granulated lymphocyte that get poured into the circulation and spread throughout the body. Some of these cells "home" for various tissues and—in their newly sequestered microenvironment—develop their secondary tissue mast cell characteristics.

Some of the P-cells that are in circulation reach the lymphatic patches located in the lower intestinal tract. These locations are known as Peyer's lymphatic patches. Here, they develop secondary characteristics that train them for their command-specific histamine-releasing roles in the mucosal tissues of the intestinal tract. They are known as mucosal mast cells when they reach their area of service.

Listen to this. In the Peyer's lymphatic patches, these immature, destined-to-be-mast-cell lymphocytes get armed with "homing receptors" and are once again poured into the circulation, determined to pass different tissue barriers until they reach their new location of service in proximity to some nerves in the gut mucosa. Before reaching the mucosa, they are lean and underdeveloped. Once they reach their destination and are in proximity to the local nerves, they become larger and develop the normal characteristics of mucosal mast cells.

The more the body gets dehydrated, the more urgently these mast cells are needed to regulate physiological functions in the body—particularly in the intestinal tract and its food-processing actions in the absence of sufficient water, with constant exposure to the bacteria and parasites that accompany food.. Every time a mast cell is forced into action, it immediately divides and produces another one like itself. In short order, one mast cell becomes two, two become four, four become eight, eight become sixteen, and so on, until the battle is won. The battle against dehydration is only won when more water enters the body and is circulated until normal physiological balance is achieved.

In old times, pigeons were used as a fast means of communication in critical circumstances. Messenger pigeons were kept well fed and protected so that their homing faculties remained efficient in case they were all of a sudden needed to go on an errand. As you might imagine, homing devices must also be efficient for man-made "robots" to become integrated into the life of any society. The same is true if they are to be used within the physiology of the body.

If you assume mast cells to be a manufacturing extension of the histamine-using nerve system at various locations in the body, then their timely arrival at the location of their service, next to the nerve system of the area, is a critical event. Their homing receptors must work flawlessly during their journey from their "cadet school for lymphocytes" to their "battlefield nerve beacons," particularly in the intestinal tract. Should a problem occur with the homing receptor before its ultimate local transformation into a mast cell, the immature lymphocyte would get stranded in the lymphatic system and become another candidate for the recycling process in the lymph glands.

Should an extraordinary crisis cause the malfunction of homing receptor proteins on all the transient immature mast cells—with the overdrive of dehydration to produce more—the outcome would be lymphatic gland engorgement with blinded mast cell lymphocytes.

T. M. Jung and associates have shown that if exposed to antigenic stimulation (possibly retroviral) at their subfinal transformation into mast cells, because of their lymphocytic properties these cells suffer the down-regulation of their homing receptors. Thus, migrant immature mast cells lose direction and the ability to reach their destination—because their homing device gets knocked out and the mast cells cannot steer toward their destination in the tissues or intestinal tract; instead, they're stranded in the blood circulation or lymphatic system.

These are natural events leading to lymphoma and leukemia production when the turbulent inner ocean of the body begins to dry up. And yet, with all the eloquence of logic and reason, diseases of the body, including its variety of cancers, will not occur unless the immune system has also gone to sleep.

DEHYDRATION AND IMMUNE SYSTEM SUPPRESSION

Dehydration, directly and indirectly, suppresses the immune system, of all places at the level of the bone marrow.

POTENT BUT INDIRECT SUPPRESSION OF THE IMMUNE SYSTEM

When histamine flexes its muscles for the regulation of the available water, along with the resources water should carry, quite a number of ruthless subagents are commissioned to modulate the events. The first thing that happens is the increased release of a chemical called vasopressin. This substance has a dual role. It immediately causes some membrane receptors to transform into porous showerhead-like sieves with holes only wide enough to let water molecules to go through the holes "single file"—one at a time, and stripped of all their other osmotically held elements.

This is a filter system designed to hydrate the most vital cells in the body—the brain cells, the liver cells, the kidney cells, the gland cells, and more. Vasopressin also creates added constrictive pressure in the area capillaries and causes forced filtration and injection of freed water from blood into the cells in its domains of operation. This mechanism delivers water into the cells by the process of reverse osmosis. This process has a price, however: It makes the consistency of blood more concentrated and thicker. The manufactured free water can now do new lifesaving work inside each cell in drought-stricken areas of the body. In the kidneys, vasopressin forces this organ to retain water and concentrate the urine.

Water filtration through cell membranes

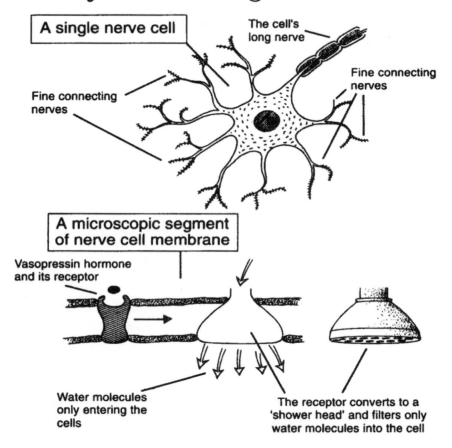

Figure 6-6. How the body selectively injects water into vital
cells through water holes created by vasopressin.
Vasopressin also increases the injection pressure
used to force water in when the blood is actually
pulling water out of the other cells in order to
supply the vital ones.

Vasopressin's function of forcing water through cell membranes is its primary role. It also has a secondary function, however: It is a very strong modulating cortisone-release factor. It influences the adrenal glands to release a number of very potent hormones—cortisol, cortisone, corticosterone, 11-deoxycorticosterone, and aldosterone—that initially prevent inflammation and also force the kidneys to retain salt 1,000 times more forcibly than normal, thereby expanding the body of water in the environment around the cells so that more can be filtered and injected into vital cells.

Cortisol and cortisone are strong anti-inflammatory agents. They exert this action by suppressing the immune system via the activation of agents such as interleukin-1. The actual damage is done when interferon production is arrested.

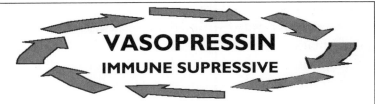

VASOPRESSIN
IMMUNE SUPRESSIVE

INCREASED CORTISONE ACTIVITY

CAUSES INTERLEUKIN-1 ACTIVELY

DEPRESSES INTERLEUKIN-2 ACTIVELY

ILK-2 STIMULATES THE IMMUNE SYSTEM
AND INTERFERON PROTECTION

ILK-1 INHIBITS THE IMMUNE SYSTEM
AND INTERFERON PROTECTION

Figure 6-7. The cortisone-releasing effects of vasopressin
ultimately result in strong immune system suppression.

Interleukin-1 is a potent immune suppressive neurotransmitter and activator of tissue breakdown. It inhibits interferon production. Why does it do all these negative things? The reason seems to be the dual roles of histamine as a water regulator and immune system activator.

When histamine engages in its water-regulating capacities—in drought—the immune system has to be disengaged; otherwise water shortage in the body would cause a flare-up of the immune system without any need for its overactivity. The role of ILK-1 in tissue breakdown is compatible with the need to release some resources from the tissues of the body—from cannibalism of the body's own tissues to the point of causing autoimmune diseases. Why does it inhibit interferon production?

In inflammatory conditions, the affected area is shut off from free flow of circulation, and thus oxygen. The swollen, inflamed region becomes overcrowded with defending white cells, to the point of pus formation: The oxygen supply from blood circulation cannot keep up with its rate of use in the center of the inflamed area. This is where interferon reveals its vital role. By acting on its receptor, interferon stimulates an enzyme that causes substantial production of ozone and hydrogen peroxide from tryptophan and its family of indolamines. These have a great affinity for storing oxygen and converting it to super-oxygens.

Hydrogen peroxide and ozone act as local antiseptics against bacteria and the anaerobic cancer cells. Some free oxygen is also provided for the stranded white cells in the middle of the inflamed and isolated area. This is how interferon normally acts as a natural and vital anticancer chemical in a properly hydrated body. In early dehydration, interferon flare-up without justification is not needed. Yet this indirect but very potent mechanism of interferon shutdown by histamine is why chronic dehydration is the primary culprit in cancer formation. The human body, under normal circumstances, has all the faculties to prevent transformed cells from becoming cancerous—but only if it does not fall into the chemical abyss of dehydration.

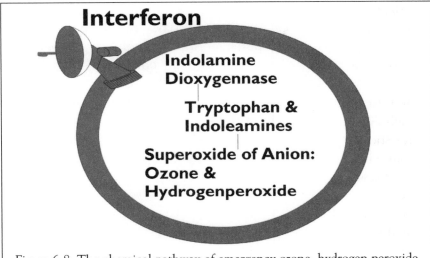

Interferon

Indolamine
Dioxygennase

Tryptophan &
Indoleamines

Superoxide of Anion:
Ozone &
Hydrogenperoxide

Figure 6-8. The chemical pathway of emergency ozone, hydrogen peroxide, and oxygen production in the areas of the body that get oxygen-depleted when the blood circulation cannot reach and deliver sufficient oxygen before angiogenesis can expand the capillary bed in the area.

The immune-suppressive action of adrenal steroids is real. As you might know, anytime there is some kind of inflammatory reaction in the body—a rash or skin eruption, say—the favorite medication of doctors is some brand of human-made cortisone, the stronger the better, but only for a very short time. Longer use of cortisone products is dangerous. It can reactivate dormant infections, such as tuberculosis, or cause ulcerations in the stomach. It causes the loss of ongoing silent battles between the immune system and offending bacteria that might want to use the available resources and establish a new home in a weakened body. Too much cortisone from outside favors intruders, and excess release of cortisone from inside can tip the edge in favor of health problems that emerge as a result of immune system suppression—such as cancer.

You now know the indirect ways the immune system becomes suppressed when the body becomes dehydrated and histamine gets engaged in the drought-management programs of the body. Let us now see how histamine inhibits the immune system, effectively and directly.

The defense system of the body depends on the precise action of its white cells. There are six different types of white cells—neutrophils, eosinophils, basophils, monocytes, lymphocytes, and plasma cells. The lymphocytic cells normally constitute about 30 percent of all white cells in the body. Most white cells, much like constantly cruising police cars, leave the blood circulation and enter into various tissues to bolster the state of local defense system; they then reenter the blood circulation via the lymphatic system. Some white cells become fixed local protective shields until used and then replaced.

Lymphocytes are mostly responsible for the manufacture of antibodies to offending agents, whereas the other white cells engage in "eating and digesting" dead and dying cells, as well as intruding elements. The antibodies from the lymphocytic line of defense attach themselves to the element that is recognized as an outsider—bacteria, viruses, parasites—and not only neutralize their toxicity but also label them for scavenging cells to devour and digest.

Like mast cells that get programmed in the lymphatic patches, the lymphocytes that need to engage in antibody formation also get programmed in the thymus gland, possibly in the liver, and definitely in the bone marrow. The ones schooled in the thymus gland are called T-cells; those from the bone marrow, B-cells. T-cell lymphocytes are divided into three subsets—helper-T-cells, cytotoxic or killer-T-cells, and suppressor-T-cells. Among them, these T-cells regulate the immune system via the chemical agents they produce, such as the interleukins (interleukin-2 to inetleukin-6), interferon, and stimulant factor for growth of the other white cells.

Histamine is also a major regulator of the complex roles of the white cells in the operation of the immune activity when there is a genuine call on the immune system. However, the system need not, and indeed must not, become activated by histamine when it engages in the drought-management programs of the body. This is how it works.

The immune system is suppressed by histamine in the bone marrow, where all the immune activity of the body originates. Suppressor T-cells are highly responsive to the action of histamine—and as it happens, there are twice as many suppressor cells as helper cells permanently residing in the bone marrow. Additionally, the suppressor T-cells in circulation also sequester to the bone marrow once stimulated by histamine. Thus, histamine puts a tight lock on the bone marrow activity through its strong influence on the larger local population of suppressor T-cells. This is how histamine prevents flare-ups of the immune system at its bone marrow origin when it gets engaged in the drought-management programs of the body.

This information has vast ramifications. Not only does it apply to the prevention of diseases such as cancer and the autoimmune disorders, but it also highlights how gradually and yet surely short-changing the body from the water it must receive daily is invitation to disaster. My latest book *Water Cures: Drugs Kill* has shown that water can reverse more than 90 major and minor health problems.

Thus there is ample justification to teach pregnant mothers and children the importance of regular intake of water to avoid immune-compromised health problems throughout life—including AIDS. I have for some time identified AIDS as a metabolic complication of unintentional dehydration, even though the outcome of its DNA fragmentation into smaller and still bioactive particles is now conveniently labeled as a worldwide viral disease. It is interesting that in Africa they have discovered that giving a multivitamin to AIDS sufferers works better than medications, at a fraction of the cost!

By now you have some understanding of how dehydration—chronic unintentional dehydration that establishes in the body when people wait until they feel thirsty to drink water, not realizing that the thirst sensation and the urge to drink water fail incrementally from age 20 onward—is the primary cause of disease, including obesity, depression, and cancer.

STEPS TO THE REMISSION OF CANCER

While the body is alive and has the will to survive, it is possible to reverse disease processes. It is not possible at present to make an old man or woman into a teenager—although that may change with the advent of cloning—but it is possible to take the aches and pains of age away and make him or her feel young again. If the body chemistry is optimized to its maximum efficiency, we can reverse some of the aging processes trumpeted by different degenerative health problems.

The body is a complex chemical plant that learns and improvises as it sees fit at any moment. It works with what you give it. Give it the right ingredients and it will purr along as it is designed to do. Give it the wrong ingredients and you force it along unchartered chemical pathways that manifest the symptoms and signs we know as disease.

When the body is given the nearest combination of the right ingredients, the symptoms and signs of normalcy—vibrant health and joyful enthusiasm—will once again shine through. This is when the disease processes go into remission. Repeat the same mistakes and you will reap the same harvest—disease. This is when cancers will also recur.

Except for infections needing antibiotics or damage to hormone-producing glands that requires replacement therapies, don't make the mistake of thinking health problems are cured by normally cytotoxic medications and chemotherapies, surgical procedures, or radiological protocols. The disease process continues if the internal chemistry of the body is not optimized by the ingredients you give it. Thus, sending cancers into remission is doable and possibly easy, but only if the right steps are taken. They are:

Attitude: If you want to live longer, do not fear death. Death is unavoidable, but if you knew how resilient the human body is, you would not fear death until it arrives. You need to rely on the survival mechanisms installed in your body. You must not give up. You need to generate the chemistry of a body that is determined to fight. With the regenerative powers of hope you will be able to direct the defense systems of your body toward survival from any naturally reversible health problem—and cancer is truly a reversible health problem. I will later give you some examples.

Meditation and prayers for reduction of stress. Unstressed people, like some who find richness in the philosophy of not wanting—the Sufi philosophy of life—live to the ripe old age of 100 or more. It is our modern-day stress, punctuated by constant frivolous needs and unneeded wants, that saddles us with this or that disease and shortens our precious lives.

Meditation and prayer connect you with the inner workings of your body, which is constantly obedient to the laws of nature and its life forces. Once you meditate or pray, the functionally quiet management side of your brain will connect to its cognitive side and generate insight into what has been wrong and why you have developed your health problem. Faith and meditation will melt away the inner fears and negative thoughts that have been eating into you. They will reverse the chemical pathways of fear; the new chemistry of salvation and repair will take over.

Love is a powerful healer—giving love or receiving it. There is an inherent insecurity that is associated with any disease, but especially cancer. When you love somebody, you want to survive to continue to be with that person. When you receive love, your body becomes energized and your immune system will lift its level of action in the fight against the disease. Love changes the chemical pathways of the brain, and this will affect your body's resistance. The love of God, for those who believe in Him, has a similar effect.

Patients are not just their "disease conditions" or "insurance add-ons"; they are vulnerable human beings. Doctors or healers must freely project their feelings of empathy and sincerity in their dealings with the sick. It is just possible their empathy might be a stronger medication than anything they might prescribe. Unfortunately medicine today suffers from the bad effects of too many get-rich-quick doctors and researchers who have entered the profession for its commercial possibilities. This is the reason we have a costly sick-care system without the ability to reverse a single health problem.

Laughter has a similar effect to love on the immune system. Periodic laughter is now being used as an additional therapeutic measure in Europe. A German lady—Barbara Rutting—who has written a book and lectures on this topic explained at a conference in Munich that the effect is associated with the attitude and posture of the face when the frown of sadness is turned into the openness of a smile. She was recommending that people laugh forcefully a number of times a day to boost their immune systems. Some group therapy sessions now include periodic laughter in their protocols.

Forgiveness has a powerful positive impact on the brain chemistry. I always use this example when I want to encourage people to forgive and forget rather than to scheme in order to avenge a hurt: Should someone undeservedly slap you in the face, if you think of his action as the result of a temporary emotional imbalance—not a reflection on you—the pain of that slap will disappear in a few minutes. However, if you take his action as a personal insult that has to be avenged, every time you think of that slap, regardless of what was your immediate reaction is at the time, the pain of the slap will come back to your face, and your brain chemistry will become engaged in that negative trip all over again. Such trips tend to consume the brain and convert its constructive powers into the negative energy of destruction.

Let me tell you about my own experience. I left my country of Iran in 1946 and entered Fettes College in Edinburgh—college used here in the English sense of the word to refer to a boarding secondary school. Five houses were used as living quarters for its 400 students. One was called Kimmergame, where my brother and I were housed. One day, when walking from the place where I did my homework to the common room at the end of the corridor, another student blocked my way! He instructed me to put up my fists. He wanted to beat the hell out of me. Even though I had a lighter skin than him, he called me a wog to justify his decision—wog is a disparaging abbreviation for "golliwog," a term for dark-skinned foreigners from the Middle East or India. He was determined to fight me. This went against my family teaching that it is a sin to hurt people, no matter how justified it may seem at the time.

I told him I did not enjoy fighting and I did not have anything against him to justify my wanting to hurt him. He did not accept this. He thought I was a coward, although I was larger and possibly stronger than him. He again commanded that I put up my fists. When I told him I did not wish to hurt him and was not going to fight, he raised his right hand and slapped me in the face with all the force he could muster. I just looked at him without any anger and asked if he had enough, offering the other side of my face in case one slap did not satisfy his hatred of people he called wogs!

He paused for a moment and all of a sudden burst into tears and began to apologize. He said what I did embodied one of Christian teachings. He did not expect such a reaction from a foreigner. He walked away repentant for having wanted to hurt me. I doubt if he was the same person after our brief encounter. Such is the power of forgiveness. I became all the stronger for conquering my anger and its direct negative effects on my brain, not only for that moment, but also through the 60 years since. Forgiving people who might have wronged you has a strong therapeutic effect. Abusive parents can psychologically scar their children for life, unless as grown-ups they learn to forgive and move on. When the children of abusive parents learn to forgive, their sicknesses, whatever they are, will mostly clear up. Hate is a truly damaging force.

Microwaves: Avoid microwave radiation: Microwave radiation, be it from high-tension lines; TV, radio, and phone towers; or cooking equipment, is not good for the body.

In the microwave oven, an electronic tube known as magnetron generates an alternating power field. Particles—water, amino acids, minerals, proteins, fat particles—in the food substance being heated are forced to align themselves in the direction of the alternating electromagnetic field. The power field that influences the oscillation of the particles changes direction up to five billion times per second. This rate of oscillation creates a considerable on–off friction rub between the particles, resulting in instant heat that affects the nutritional value of the food.

David Broom, a herbalist and a Kirlian photographer—Hurn Forest Clinic, 40 Wayside Road, St. Leonard, Hants, England—has done some telling photography of microwaved foods. Kirlian photos record the aura of energy emitted by living matter. Carrots that are organically raised have a very intense aura of energy. Microwave them only for five seconds and you lose much of their life energy. The same is true for mushrooms (see figure 6-9) and other foods. If the body is trying to capture the life energy in a piece of carrot, microwaving it will reduce the advantage of eating the carrot. Just imagine what happens to the frozen food that is prepared to satisfy the people who wish to eat and watch television!

Fresh vs Microwave Mushroom

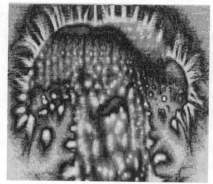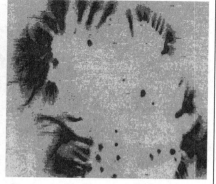

Figure 6-9. A mushroom before and after five seconds of microwave heating. The mushroom on the left is full of life energy that the Kirlian camera can record. On the right, the same mushroom is shown with almost no life-energy that the body could benefit from after 5 seconds of microwave heating. Reprinted by kind permission of David Broom, from his book The Life in Your Food: As Seen Through Kirlian Photography.

Microwaves have carcinogenic effects on the human body, regardless of the number of times the authorities have tried to deny this fact. I attended the World Foundation for Natural Science conference in 1999 in Lindau, Germany. A number of scientists, including Dr. Hans U. Hertel of The World Foundation for Natural Science, one of the foremost scientists in this field, spoke about the hazards of microwaves for people who were constantly exposed to them. One of the speakers from a European university had done an experiment that left a deep imprint on me. He left no doubt in my mind that people should avoid having anything to do with microwaves in their environment!

He had taken a piece of liver and divided it into two sections. One section he studied under a microscope, recording normal liver cell structures. The other section was microwaved via a rod pushed inside its tissue. The slides from the second section showed a total disruption of the liver cell architecture. The cytoplasm of the cells had become mushy, and all the solid particles had separated and grouped together in a linear fashion. Different mineral elements had separated from their attachments and were grouped together, calcium with calcium, sodium with sodium, and so on, as if they'd been centrifuged.

This experiment convinced me that we should avoid persistent exposure to microwaves at any cost. It is true that no one is going to stick a microwave rod inside our body for a quick kill, but long-term microwave exposure, such as the constant use of cell phones, must have a similar effect on any tissue it can reach. After I came back from that conference, we got rid of the microwave oven we had at home, although we very seldom used it. The moral of this story: If you want to stay healthy or wish to recover from a disease, cancer in particular, eat fresh food; if you prefer to cook it, use regular convection heat. By nature, I am not an alarmist, but I am alarmed myself about the use of microwaves.

Water: They are wrong when they say that after oxygen, water is the most important substance for life. Water is more important.

After all, if there were no water, oxygen would not be able to reach the inner workings of cells. It is true that oxygen is used in the composition of water, but as a primary substance, water is more important for prevention and cure of all sorts of health problems, from heartburn to cancer.

You have to prudently prevent dehydration. Contrary to the recent recommendation—obviously uninformed about advances in physiologic understanding of dehydration—of the Food and Nutrition Panel of the National Academy of Sciences, you must not wait to get thirsty in the traditional sense of developing a dry mouth before you drink. Dry mouth is not an accurate indicator of early, but nonetheless pathology-producing, thirst. At the same time, you must not exaggerate and drink too much water. You will wash out some of your body's precious minerals unnecessarily, to the point of causing brain damage. Try to stick to the water–salt formula given in the last chapters of this book. A good indicator is the color of your urine: Drink enough that urine fluctuates between perceptibly light yellow and colorless.

For the treatment of skin cancers, repeated bathing and hot-water massage of the cancer tissue may prove very effective. You need to bring more circulation to the base of skin to fight the cancer cells. Hot water will help. I got to know a Princeton professor who told me about his experience with an extensive ulcerating melanoma of his back. After he could not get any relief from his treatments in one of the teaching hospitals in Philadelphia, he instinctively decided to stay in his bathtub for two hours a day and soak his back with warm water. He would sometimes use some mineral salts in the water. He cured his own cancer in this way.

I met a lady at my first lecture—Cancer: Another Cry for Water—at the Cancer Control Society conference in San Diego in 1994. She had a very large cancer at the back of her left hand. She had decided to attend one of the famous clinics in California that use lifestyle and nutrition changes to treat disease. She wanted to know my opinion and if she could do anything more to get rid of her cancer. I told her to drink water and to soak her hand in warm water as often as she could daily. The institution she attended did not advocate water consumption. Its staff believed only in "juicing" the body. I ran into this woman again in 2002, at the same conference in Los Angeles. She told me her cancer had healed very rapidly after she used water internally as well as bathing her hand in warm water. Here is the why of it.

Skin Circulation in Dehydration

The structure of skin is made up of several layers. There is an external, compacted dying-cells layer that is exposed to the elements outside the body. Immediately beneath this compacted layer is the layer of vibrantly lively skin cells that constantly grow and replace the external layer, which peels off and gets scraped because of friction. Then, under the actively growing layer, is a layer of fatty deposits that act as a shock absorber and heat and cold insulator for the structures beneath it, such as muscle tissue and superficial bones. Two layers of capillary circulation can serve the skin. One layer is located between the skin layer and fat under it. Another mesh of capillaries is found under the fat layer, just over the muscle tissue. These two meshworks are interconnected by branches that traverse the fatty layer, figure 6-10.

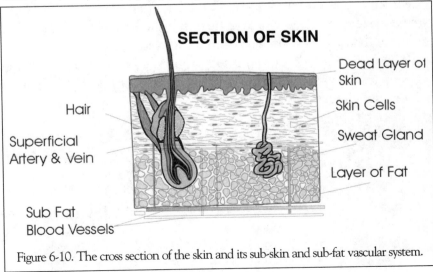

Figure 6-10. The cross section of the skin and its sub-skin and sub-fat vascular system.

When we are young and the cells of the body are well hydrated, blood circulation in the outermost mesh of capillaries serves the skin, because the body has enough water reserves to afford its constant loss to the atmosphere—hence the rosy color of the skin in the young. As we age and our perception of thirst becomes less acute, permitting the body to become unintentionally dehydrated, the outer capillary bed is closed down more and more. The subfatty layer of capillaries provides some blood circulation to the skin cells, but hardly enough to compensate for the constant loss of water from the skin—hence the gray, furrowed, dehydrated skin in the elderly.

Proper hydration by mouth—including the restoration of the salt and mineral reserves of the body—opens up the capillary circulation in the subskin layer. The heat from hot-water immersion of the skin stimulates the nerve endings in the area. They cause the immediately subskin capillary bed to open up and supply the water needed for perspiration and sweating to cool the body. In the process, some toxic waste is also excreted through the sweat glands.

Thus, as a treatment protocol for skin cancers, hot water serves a dual purpose. First, the skin sensors also let the brain know that water is available and that its rationing programs—which shut down surface circulation to the skin in the first place—need not be strictly executed. Second, the heat supplied by water causes the capillary bed to open up and bring more water, oxygen, raw materials, and energized immune cells to the base of the cancerous growth in the skin, a natural and effective treatment protocol for superficial cancers.

> **Note:** To deal with cancer tissue, the body has to bring more circulation to the area. Since the insufficiency of microcirculation and low oxygen flow are the primary trigger mechanisms for cancer transformation of local cells, correction of the problem is the first step toward repairing the damage. Toward this end, the local vascular bed of capillaries will need to expand, and new blood vessels be formed.

The process is known as angiogenesis. Commercial medicine, always looking for a moneymaking angle, has presented the body's natural defense mechanism of forming more blood vessels to fight disease as something the cancer cells do to grow. They have tried to produce chemicals to prevent angiogenesis, with results that are, as far as I have heard, catastrophic. Such treatments should be avoided. Hydrate and make the body alkaline to fully activate its defense systems. Let the body deal with the problem naturally and without commercial interference.

Minerals: A balance of minerals in the diet is crucial to prevention of cancer. It becomes even more critical for the treatment of cancers. You need salt to expand the volume of blood in circulation so that it stays dilute and reaches all the nooks and crannies of the body. Salt will also help make the inside of the cells of the body alkaline, essential for preventing and treating cancer. The other mineral components of unrefined salt—calcium, magnesium, potassium, selenium, zinc, and up to 80 other trace elements—expand the water content of the cell interior and make it alkaline. Thus, unrefined sea salt, or unrefined salt from land deposits, must be used instead of regular table salt that has been stripped of its vitally important companion minerals. There is more information on minerals in the final chapters of this book.

Green vegetables: Green is good for you. Chlorophyll contains much magnesium, in the same way hemoglobin contains much iron. They are both oxygen carriers. Chlorophyll has the effect of making the body alkaline. Green vegetables contain many vital elements needed to sustain life—vitamins, minerals, proteins, essential fats, antioxidants, and phytochemicals. If you get uncomfortable eating bulky vegetables, you can always juice them.

Fruits: Colorful fruits and berries have many antioxidant properties. They make the body alkaline. Fresh fruits prevent free-radical
damage. The body can meet many of its mineral needs, such as
those for potassium and calcium, via fruit. Bananas, citrus fruits,
mango, pineapple, tomatoes—I consider tomato a fruit akin to passion fruit, which grows on a vine, too—apples, plums, peaches, avocado, melons, and more, are God's medications for a sick body, especially for a cancer-stricken body. Juice them or eat them as they
come, but make sure you have several helpings of them every day.

Let me tell you my story. I was ten years old when I developed
typhoid fever and became semiconscious. There was an epidemic of
the fever at the time; many thousands had fallen sick from a con-
taminated drinking water source. In those days there were no
antibiotics. Proper loving care and good nursing were the only ways
to tip the balance in favor of survival in a resilient body. My daily
diet included several glasses of "sweet lemon" juice. It took me five
months to overcome the fever and achieve full consciousness. Many
thousands could not make it and died. My mother's loving attention
and the daily lemon juice she forced me to take helped me survive.
They were my natural immune-system-boosting medications.

Proteins with a balanced amino acid composition: Proteins are essential as building blocks for the physical structures of the body. They are
also used for the manufacture of enzymes, receptors, and neurotransmitters in the brain. This topic is discussed fully in the last chapters of the
book. Proteins tend to make the body acidic. This is why there should
be a balance between the amount of fruits and vegetables in the diet
and your protein intake. An ideal composition is around 80 percent
fruits, vegetables (roots like carrots, beet root, turnip, potato, and sweet
potato have high mineral content), and legumes, which are high in protein and ideally balanced in amino acids. Legumes, such as lentils, fava
beans—also known as broad beans—chickpeas, green beans, and soybeans, are about 28 percent protein. Only 20 percent of the protein in
the diet should be from other sources—meat, fish, fowl, eggs, and
cheese, particularly cottage cheese, which is rich in the amino acid tryptophan. Turkey breast is also rich in tryptophan, whereas beef is not.

Exercise is one of the physiological pedestals on which life stands. It helps blood circulate into all corners of the body, hydrate and oxygenate each region, and preserve local health. Proper regional hydration and oxygenation of tissues are sure steps to cancer prevention. Exercise is vital for efficient lymphatic flow back to the heart. Muscle contraction exerts pumping pressure and forces the lymph to flow in the lymphatic vessels upward and onward to reach the heart and get mixed with blood to be circulated again. Exercise will direct the body physiology toward conservation of tryptophan and the other essential amino acids, vital for prevention of cancer.

Sunlight, and its subset of light systems, reaches and stimulates the special sensors on the skin of the face and the forehead, as well as the light sensors of the eye. These energy fields of light program and set the biological clock of the body to naturally integrate the hormonal secretion of its glands. Sunlight is a healing energy. It helps correct osteoporosis and the soft-bone complications of rickets in children. Sunlight converts cholesterol to vitamin D and encourages storage of ATP energy in the calcium deposits within the cells of the body—a vital step in boosting the immune activity of the body.

Music: Masaru Emoto, M.D., an outstanding Japanese scientist, has introduced a new topic into the science of medicine. He has discovered that water is influenced both by what it "hears" and by the toxins that pollute it. Ernoto has demonstrated this phenomenon by influencing water with sound, or taking water from sources that already contain toxins, and then freezing that water until it forms ice crystals. Classical and harmonious music produces clear, smooth ice crystals. Loud heavy-metal music produces abnormal or deformed crystals. The ice from water that contains toxins, such as dioxin, produces abnormal and deformed ice crystals. Even kind or unkind words such as thank you or devil written on the glass influence the shape and texture of the ice crystals.

"Love and thankfulness show the most beautiful crystals in the world," Ernoto reports. Mozart, Bach, and Chopin produced different variations on "happy ice crystals." These experiments leave no room for doubt that water reacts to what it hears. Remember, the body is about 75 percent water; the influence of harmonious sound can thus translate into the inner harmony of our body with the powers of nature in us, exerting a strong healing influence. Happiness-generating music should be used in the treatment protocol of any disease, particularly as an effective natural process in cancer treatment.

Note: There is a belief among some scientists that water retains the memory of its past encounters. Dr. Benveniste of INSERM in France is the person who, based on some experiments in his laboratory, first announced the discovery, which was later discredited by *Nature* in its July 28, 1988 publication. In November of 1989 I wrote to Dr. Benveniste and showed him where his experiment was faulty and why his conclusions were erroneous. You could read my published letter among the scientific articles at www.watercure.com. Dr. Emoto's findings about the influence of sound on water may be used to wrongly resurrect Dr. Benveniste's erroneous claims. At a conference in Munich in October of 2003, where Dr. Emoto and I were speakers, I asked him, if the ice with "influenced" shapes melt and that water is frozen again, does it retain the memory of what had influenced it the first time, and does it reproduce the modified shape? His reply was "it does not." This proves that it is wrong to claim water retains the memory of its past encounters.

Humanitarian undertakings—better still if they are faith-based—program the brain into a purposeful, constructive mode of life. Such activities take you away from constant thoughts of yourself and focus some of your brain's energy expenditure on altruism. This produces a sense of fulfillment that has a positive effect on the physiology of the brain and can reverse the stress of life. Undertakings based on genuine empathy have a healing effect on the brain. This seems to be the reason for the highlight of the Masonic charge to the apprentice Masons: "Blessed is he who gives as well as him who receives."

How Some Cancers Were
Reversed by Water

I would like to begin with Andrew J. Bauman IV. His malignant melanoma and lymphoma were the outcome of a number of years of symptom-producing dehydration. His first symptoms of dehydration began with allergies at the age of eight. He also had some breathing problems associated with his allergies. At 14 he developed diabetes—one of the harshest of the drought-management programs of the body. By 23 his asthma needed treatment for him to stay alive. At 26 he developed diabetic neuropathy affecting his eyesight and circulatory problems in his feet and legs.

From the age of 20 onward, he had many bouts of glandular fever, indicating that his immune system was being suppressed.

Andrew Bauman, age 42

- **Allergies: age 8**
- **Astma needing tretament: age 23**
- **Diabetes: age 14**
- **Immune System Suppression: age 20**
- **Neuropathy: age 26**
- **Lump skin left flank: Biopsy Sept. 1995**
  Lymphoma
    Gallium test result :
    Lymphoma all over the body

- **"Water Cure" November 1995**
- **Gallium test result: March 1996**
  No Cancer Cells Anywhere

Figure 6-10. The sequence of dehydration symptoms that eventually culminated in lymphoma.

Note: I use Drew's full name in the letter that follows to leave no doubt that such a person does exist. He lives in New York and is now studying Chinese medicine. Drew Bauman's history of illness is unique in the way it illustrates the sequence of physiological events that takes place when the body becomes persistently dehydrated. When you read the letter, you will begin to realize the connection between so many disease conditions and gradually establishing dehydration, and the emerging connection of major health issues to one another.

In Drew's case, the dehydration of early childhood revealed itself in the form of allergies and proceeded to manifest as diabetes, asthma, immune suppression and repeated infections, vascular disease, and eventually cutaneous B-cell lymphoma. He had to go from one doctor to another and one hospital to another for the symptomatic treatment of his various health problems. Ultimately, his treatment included being X-ray-roasted, and he sustained extensive burns. Until he refused further treatment, they wanted to continue his X-ray-roasting to kill his cancer cells. Fortunately, he realized that he would die more quickly from his treatment protocol than from his variety of health problems.

In April 2003, I received an elated call from Drew. He had undergone extensive examination and investigation to see if he is still cancer-free. He got a clean bill of health. His "traditional" doctors were flummoxed and wanted to know how he had done it. Apparently, it is unheard of for his kind of lymphoma not to recur in six years. He proceeded to explain to them the WaterCure protocol! In August 2004, I am happy to report that Drew is very well and extremely successful at preaching the WaterCure wherever he can.

Let me also explain why Drew was contracting so many infections. Histamine is the primary water regulator of the body. It is also a primary immune system regulator. But when histamine gets engaged in water regulation of the body, it automatically suppresses the immune system at its bone marrow level of activity. It has to do it; otherwise dehydration would constantly cause immune system flare-up. This is the natural design of the body to conserve the immune system for serious infections and not waste its resources when the body is dehydrated.

Dear Dr. Batmanghelidj,

My name is Andrew J. Bauman IV, and I am 42 years young, yet at
age 34 I felt and looked like I was at least 44! Most of my life has been
spent battling illness and disease, whereas now I celebrate each
moment of each day with a renewed vigor and vitality. I used to be
chronically dehydrated and now I know better.

I was born on October 29, 1956, in Taylor, PA, in a small hospital
near Scranton in northeast Pennsylvania. My parents lovingly cared for
me—including having me vaccinated. I was reared on infant formula
and later cereal, juices, and a small amount of water when I would cry
from colic. After my first polio vaccine, I became mysteriously para-
lyzed from the waist down. Specialists were puzzled, yet diagnosed
"aborted polio." It left as suddenly as it appeared. When I received a
booster dose of the vaccine at around age 5 in first grade, the paralysis
returned. Months of hospitalization and bed rest resulted in my gaining
weight. I mostly ate my meals and had visitors, drank soda, and some
water now and then—and once again the paralysis disappeared.

When I began third grade—around eight years old—my allergic afflictions
and symptoms had begun. I had problems with frequent dry coughs. I
began experiencing some difficulties with breathing, itchy and watery eyes,
and fatigue when I was around fresh-cut lawns from springtime until
autumn. When I was a junior in high school, I experienced blackouts
from allergies. Sometime around 1979, I saw a specialist who did testing
and diagnosed me with allergies and asthma. I was approximately 23
years old. I was treated with allergy shots and inhalers. The treatments
just seemed to make things worse. My lips were always dry and cracked.
At that time of my life I was drinking about 2 to 4 cups of coffee per day
along with a few glasses of soda and some tea and alcohol. I would have
an occasional glass of water during the day. The allergies and asthma
stayed with me until 1996 when my water intake was up to about two to
three quarts a day. I no longer struggle with allergies or asthma.

My problems with diabetes began at age 14. I was diagnosed as an
insulin-dependent or "juvenile diabetic." It was then that I began drink-

ing diet beverages including those with caffeine. My water intake at that time was still only around 2 to 4 glasses a day and I was drinking tea and started drinking coffee. The diabetes resulted in many hospitalizations over the years. By the mid-1980s I had problems with diabetic neuropathy that was causing my legs to swell. I was scheduled to have dye injected into my legs to perform a diagnostic scan after a Doppler radar study showed some apparent blockages in the veins on my legs. The dye injections caused my veins to burst, which made the swelling worse. I was then diagnosed with "venous insufficiency." In 1994, I was told that my legs would probably have to be amputated within a year or so.

While attempting to get on a diabetic insulin supply trial, the initial examination revealed that the retinas in my eyes had grown blood vessels that were bleeding (diabetic retinopathy). I began receiving a series of laser surgeries over the next 15 years to attempt to seal the leaky vessels and to attempt to prevent any new vessel growth. This reduced my peripheral and night vision. In 1992, I developed an enlarged yet benign prostate gland and my kidneys began showing signs of deterioration. In 1993, I began experiencing some potency difficulties. In 1994, I began seeing a natural or homeopathic physician who, besides treating me with alternative medicine, advised me to increase my water intake. My intake of insulin was around 95 units of insulin daily.

In 1976, many immune system problems began developing. I graduated from high school in 1974 and went away to college. In 1976, I got a job as a mental health worker while going to school. I met my wife and while dating, working full time, and going to school part time, I developed "infectious mononucleosis." My wife and I were married in 1977, and I continued to struggle with many infections and illnesses as well as losing my job in 1978. In 1979, during one of my then frequent hospital stays, I was diagnosed with "mono" again! The doctors insisted that I shouldn't have it again and began consulting with specialists. I received an influenza vaccine and was discharged; only to be readmitted one day later with a fever of 106°F. I was undergoing many tests, however nothing much was showing up at that time. After many tests for severe abdominal pain, I was told that I grew a second spleen that was attached to my spleen and that the second one was also functioning. That year I was visiting someone, and drank unpasteurized milk and ended up in the hospital again with a bacterial infection of the intestinal tract. "Brucellosis and proteus—ox-19" was the diagnosis and I was on yet more antibiotics.

During 1980 or 1981, I developed another case of "mono" and was admitted to the hospital again; diabetic control problems were a constant battle for me. An infectious disease specialist discovered that a number of special antibodies against foreign agents were also affected, which the doctors suggested were related to the problems with my allergies and asthma, as well as my frequent infections.

The 1980s were filled with many hospitalizations, illnesses, job losses, and stress-related problems. It was then that I was diagnosed with allergies to penicillin and tetracycline, began developing hypertension, was diagnosed with chronic fatigue syndrome, lymphoid hyperplasia (overstressed immune system), arthritis, bursitis, fibromyalgia, gastroparesis or acid reflux problems, and bowel problems. I also developed a benign tumor on the left flank of my back. I developed a nodule on my thyroid area and was diagnosed with lead, cadmium, and aluminum poisoning, which were also found in a landfill I lived near. I was overweight and developed sleep apnea. Tests showed that I stopped breathing over 300 times in a six-hour period and had "narcolepsy." I could fall asleep in a short period of time. I had surgery to attempt to correct the sleep apnea, and I wore a tracheotomy tube in my neck to help me breathe at night, and slept with a breathing machine to keep my airway open. During the '80s I still only drank a few glasses of water, yet consumed large amounts of coffee, saccharine, and eventually NutraSweet. In 1987, I was declared "disabled"!

In 1992, at 36 years old, I looked and felt like I was in my late forties and felt worse than I looked. I began using natural supplements with vitamins, herbs, and other natural medical techniques. The natural doctor's advice was to increase my water consumption and decrease my caffeine intake as well. I had lost the feeling in my feet, was always tired and achy, depressed, and had little hope.

I began to drink more water and reduced my caffeine intake somewhat and by 1995, I began to feel and look much better. Yet I was still only consuming a quart to a quart and a half daily, and not flushing all the caffeine out of my system, nor was I using sea salt.

In September of 1995 that lump on my left flank turned red, and began itching and enlarging. My family physician removed it and sent it away for study. In October, I was diagnosed with cutaneous B-cell lymphoma. Twenty-six new tumors had grown on my back where there was one and I was sent to a major hospital where I was told that lymphatic cancer on the skin surface was rare and that not much research was done yet on it. I went for a gallium test and it revealed that my entire body surface glowed positive for cancer cells. The flank of my back was brighter white or "hyperpositive," as was the middle of my chest where two melanomas were previously removed. I was advised to receive localized radiation and as tumors appeared we would radiate them too or I could travel to Philadelphia and have my entire body surface radiated. They began to radiate my back, which began giving me third-degree burns. I refused total body radiation and midway through my radiation my homeopathic physician began using a natural cleansing therapy. The cancer specialist had advised me to try anything and to "pull out all the stops as well as to get my affairs in order." I increased my water consumption and took supplements and natural treatments.

In November of 1995, while traveling in search of an answer, I had to buy tires for my car. At the auto parts store where I was looking for tires, I was introduced to Bob Butts who exposed me to your WaterCure program and advised me to stick to it very seriously to get cured. I now began to seriously increase my water intake but was still leery of increasing salt intake due to the traditional medical contra-indications for its perceived high blood pressure problems. Later, I learned of the error of that thinking and began to increase my salt intake too. In March of 1996, I went for another gallium scan, which revealed that there was not a single sign of cancer glowing positive on my entire body. Doctors thought there was an error in the gallium scan, but my homeopath and I knew that I was healing. Drinking more water, reducing caffeine, and change in dietary habits, natural medicine, and faith had brought me home. I acknowledge God's presence in me and remember the scripture, "I am the living waters." He called you and me "the salt of the earth," and tells us that we are "one in spirit."

Since then I've been constantly improving in my health. I no longer have two spleens, but one that is normal in size and function. Now I lick sea salt off my palm in the morning before my first glass of water and use salt liberally. I drink about 1.5 gallons of water a day and take some supplements as well as eating a lot of whole grains, and fresh fruits and vegetables. My waist used to be a size 40 and now is a size 36. I weighed 249 pounds, now I weigh 210 and have solid muscle mass. My complexion and appearance are those of a man in his early thirties and my potency of a man in his twenties. My ankles are no longer swollen and new pulses, yes new pulses have developed where once they were dead. I no longer take any medications for all those problems, whereas I used to be on at least 15 prescriptions at a time. My insulin needs are down from 95 units a day to 35–45 units a day. I no longer suffer with "chronic infections" or fatigue—I sleep 6–8 hours a day instead of 12–14. It is rare for me to take antibiotics, whereas I seemed to be constantly taking them before. I don't have allergies or asthma or gastroparesis (acid reflux) anymore. I no longer suffer from arthritis, bursitis, or bowel problems. At the time of my last stress test, my doctor who is younger than I am told me that I was in better shape than he was. The high blood pressure is constantly improving. No more thyroid nodule, I sleep better, and no more heavy metal toxicity. I have a new lease on life.

My prayers have been answered. God led me to a natural way to heal my body, my mind, and my spirit. I am living a new life now with a balance of water, salt, minerals, supplements, good nutrition, and continued improvements in my quality of life. I am truly blessed.
You have my permission to use this letter in any way you think will help spread the news of the medicinal value of water in medical treatment procedures.

Sincerely, Andrew J. Bauman, IV

You were given scientific information on lymphocytes—precursor cells to histamine-producing white cells—and how they can lose their way and get stranded in the lymphatic system when there is dehydration. In Drew Bauman's letter you discover how correcting dehydration and its complications can reverse this pathology. I do hope people in cancer research will use the information and not discard it because they want to protect our present commerce-friendly hocus-pocus way of practicing medicine.

I sincerely think it is possible to prevent lymphomas all the time. If people apply the information I have provided in this book, I expect that more than 95 percent of full-blown lymphomas will go into remission with the same protocol. We may need to fine-tune the protocol with further research to identify other minor elemental and mineral deficiencies and achieve 100 percent remission rates.

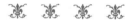

Dear Dr. Batmanghelidj,

Several months ago I finished reading your fascinating book Your Body's Many Cries for Water. I truly have to say that I couldn't put it down until I finished reading it. Several of my friends and family members have also read it. My brother, who has some medical background, has also read it, and he found it very interesting.

I have a medical condition called polycythemia vera. My body produces too many red blood cells. I am on medication called hydroxyurea. Also from time to time they have to do a phlebotomy on me. I was diagnosed with this illness about nine years ago when I was 33 years old, but my doctor said that probably I had the illness several years before that. It is a rare illness usually occurring in much older people. People of my age usually do not have this illness. Nobody knows what causes this illness. I was told perhaps stress has something to do with it. Also, I used to be a security guard for several years and I worked in factories and industrial sites and perhaps I was exposed to some chemicals or toxic materials. Over the years my condition seemed to get slightly worse. I was put on hydroxyurea. The use of hydroxyurea over an extended period of time can lead in some cases to leukemia and other illnesses.

About eight months ago I read your book and I started drinking more water. I drink about 80 ounces a day. Over the years I have also suffered from hypertension and I was under a lot of pressure from my doctor to go on high blood pressure medication. At first my blood pressure was borderline, but it seemed to be getting worse. I resisted as long as I could about taking the high blood pressure medication, but I don't think that I could have resisted much longer. I started drinking 80 ounces of water a day eight months ago. Now my blood pressure is totally normal. As a matter of fact, during my last checkup one of the nurses joked that I have the blood pressure of a teenager.

As far as my polycythemia vera is concerned there has also been an improvement. As I mentioned above my condition seemed to be getting slightly worse. I started drinking more water eight months ago. Now my condition seems to be improving. Every three months or so, I go for a checkup and each time they take a sample of my blood for laboratory tests. Among the things they test for, my brother told me, is something called RDW. As best as I can explain what my brother has told me, RDW shows how healthy my cells are, whether they have mutated or not. If they mutate enough, this can lead to leukemia and other medical conditions. This RDW measurement had also been getting slightly worse. The RDW number is now totally normal.

Soon I will ask my doctor whether gradually I can be taken off the medication and rely more on phlebotomy. Both my doctor and my brother have talked about me doing this.

I have described as best as I could both of my medical conditions and how by drinking more water they have both improved significantly. It is a shame that the medical establishment does not take the drinking of larger amounts of water more seriously. I only wish I would have known about all of this many years ago. I do know that I will tell all my friends and relatives about this. I wish I could do much more in helping you promote your theories.

With my best wishes, I remain

Sincerely, Ivan

The two most deadly cancers are prostate cancer in men and breast cancer in women. These two seem to respond to the immune-system-activating effects of water. Let me first explain prostate cancer; then I will discuss the cancer of the breast.

The prostate gland has an enzyme system that is responsive to increased acidity in its environment. Once the enzyme acid phosphatase gets activated, it begins to promote protein formation and the enlargement of the tissues around it. Thus, persistent dehydration and low acid clearance from the body are the primers for the hypertrophy of the prostate gland. Correcting dehydration and making the body alkaline can reverse the process. Here is one example. Please note that the process will also alleviate other problems.

Prostate Cancer

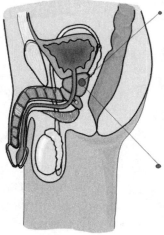

• Prostate gland enlarges and enventually developes cancer when its tissue becomes more and more acidic.

• It has high levels of **"acid phosphatase"** enzymes which promote growth in acidic medium

Figure 6-11. Why the prostate gland is prone to enlargement and cancer when the body becomes acidic.

Dear Dr. B,

I recently read your book Your Body's Many Cries for Water and I have seriously been following your advice since the first of January, drinking 8–10 glasses of water per day.

Three things have happened to me physically since I started following your advice. First the prostate problems that I have had for more than eight years seem to be getting much, much better. As you can see I live in a high, dry place. Prior to your book I could not sleep through the night because of the dryness in my nose and mouth. Now, I have no problems. Finally, the fungus that I have had under my toenails since the Korean War is gone!

I know many more important things have been reported to you, but these were important to me. I appreciate all the work you're doing.

Regards, R. D. B.

Note: The fungus disappeared because R. D. B.'s immune system was released from its inhibited state. This enabled it to deal with the fungus as well as any early cancer transformation in the prostate tissue itself.

WATER AND SALT
CURED PROSTATE CANCER

July 1999, routine test - PSA 4.6
Biopsy confirmed tumor

January 2000, PSA 5.7
Walter Reed Medical Center

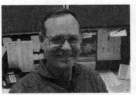

Chose hydration to radiation,
chemotherapy, seeding or surgery

Wells Jackson
61 years old

January 2001, PSA Reduced to 3.5
Walter Reed Medical Center Confirmed remission

Figure 6-12. The steps in diagnosis of prostate cancer and its remission through water intake.

Dear Dr. Batmanghelidj:

I am writing to thank you for leading me through the cure of prostate cancer.

During a flight physical in July 1999 my PSA was at 4.6. I was referred to a urologist; that led to a biopsy, which came back positive in October. I went to Walter Reed Medical Center for a second opinion in January 2000 where my PSA was found to be at 5.7 and it was confirmed as cancer.

While home for Christmas, my mother kept talking about your book Your Body's Many Cries for Water. I finally asked her to please stop talking about it so I could enjoy the holidays and my granddaughters, but I promised to read the material she gave me on the flight back to Germany. While I was at Walter Reed in Washington, D.C., I found out all I could about possible cures and facilities or clinics that might serve as alternative resources, because everyone I talked to wanted to operate. Actually, three choices were recommended to me: wait and watch, radiation therapy, and surgery, which was their strongest recommendation.

I began drinking water while at Walter Reed as a result of downloading your volumes of information from the Internet at www.watercure.com. I e-mailed you because I had some questions, and when I returned to Europe I found an answer from you inviting me to call you at your office, which I did. You asked me many questions and told me to begin drinking water, carrot juice, and orange juice, use salt (which I had not done for twenty years), eat lots of vegetables and fruits and the only eating restriction you gave me was to not eat fried foods. You also told me to give up coffee, alcohol, and sodas. You told me to walk for an hour in the morning and an hour at night, faithfully. You invited me to call you whenever I had questions and when I asked what it would cost, you stated there would be no charge . . . WOW!!!

Since then I have called regularly, every week at first and about once a month more recently. I have had monthly PSA tests run and they generally have been within safe tolerance since February (the first month after beginning the WaterCure). In March I went to Panama and Vietnam and was not able to follow the regime faithfully but I did keep drinking my daily amount of water and my PSA was slightly elevated when it was tested in April. I went back to the regime and the PSA was way down the next month.

I went to Panama for a family reunion in late July and early August, where I drank some beer and coffee and when I returned to Europe I found my PSA was up again. This concerned me and I called to speak with you about it. In our conversation you questioned me very closely about the consumption of alcohol and I confessed that since I live in Germany where the world's best beers are available, I usually had one or two at dinner. You told me not to drink any alcohol and I obeyed. You also shared with me that the high PSA indicated a higher acidity in my body and recommended that I eat lots of vegetables, particularly green ones, to cause a higher pH. The next month's test was at 3.3.

At first when I attempted to explain what I am doing to medical doctors they basically blew me off, but more recently I have spoken to a few who are interested. Since beginning this suggested regime, I have really felt better than before I started. I was in pretty good shape, but within three weeks, I noticed that when I did the same cardiovascular exercises as before, I had to work much harder to raise my heartbeat to the normal 150 that I had always achieved before. It would only reach 130 with the same effort. I asked you about this and you told me it was because my heart muscles were probably dehydrated before and no longer have to work so hard. With the same effort now, I only achieve a heart rate of 115 to 120.

For years I have had some pains in my knees and in one hip when I walked or ran and my knees hurt when I walked after getting up out of a chair . . . This was completely gone after about three months of water drinking. My nagging lower back pain has disappeared and I really feel great. I am 60 and quite frankly I feel about as good as I did at 40 and I am cured of prostate cancer.

I was raised on a farm, flew fighters, built houses and commercial buildings, and owned a number of construction consulting businesses in my adult years, so from my experience I am a practical thinker and water makes sense. I can personally claim that your information works and it is amazing that so many other friends of mine think it is just too simple a solution. It is particularly distressing to encounter the ignorance shown by traditional medical people who seem to be blinded by their training and professional arrogance when it comes to acceptance of your information. Thank you very much Dr. Batmanghelidj and I pray that "WE" are successful in getting your practical information heard by people who can benefit from it.

Please feel free to share this information with anyone it will benefit.

Respectfully, W. J.

Note: Mr. Jackson went back to the Walter Reed Medical Center the following year for reevaluation of his condition. All the tests done on him were negative for cancer. He was told to do another checkup in a year. He has been clear of cancer since then.

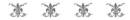

Dear Dr. Batmanghelidj,

You will appreciate that Ken and I were not so much concerned with constructing a clinical record as we were with bringing to Ken's diagnosis of advanced, untreatable prostate cancer every healing resource that we could muster. I've reconstructed the events as best as I can from supplier invoices, Medicare documents, physicians' bills, and so forth. I'm also enclosing a photocopy of the lab reports developed from blood drawings and urine samples in Houston, TX.

PSA readings on June 4 and July 9 and the biopsy taken on July 9 certainly confirm Dr. Syperd's recommendations that Ken should forgo any kind of treatment and expect to die within 18 months of the prostate cancer. I ordered your books, videotapes, and audiotapes on July 6 and likely received them about July 14. I ordered ConcenTrace on July 13 and probably received it about July 21.

No doubt at all exists that Ken's experience with increased water intake began after the second PSA reading (50.8) was taken. In my recollection Ken began the regimen the day after your book and videotapes were received. For five days Ken's urine was such a dark brown and so dankly smelly that we were alarmed. "It's the cancer cells being expelled," I encouraged him. Ken was sweating profusely and with an acrid, repellent odor. He had to change his bed linens and his clothes (after a shower) several times a day. Ken was drinking from 11 to 13 glasses (8 oz water in a 10 oz glass) of home-distilled water each day. He began each day as you suggested with two glasses of water. Abruptly in the mid afternoon of the fifth day, Ken's urine appeared clear and his sweating diminished and returned to its ordinary odor.

Exactly when Ken began adding ConcenTrace to our home-distilled water I can't be certain. Ken didn't like the taste of 30 drops/gallon and for a few days he experimented with the amount, finally settling on 18 drops/gallon.

Ever since we purchased the home distiller from Sears several years ago I've been nagging him to enhance the water with minerals. In 1967 I had collapsed with clinical depression, which in 1970 was attributed to a gross calcium/magnesium imbalance resulting from my drinking water treated by a Culligan water softener. Since those days, I've been dedicated to mineral supplements. Ken, however, had done nothing to replace the minerals lost by distilling our water.

When the pretreatment PSA report came back to the Burzynski Clinic in Houston, Ken was asked how his PSA could have dropped so dramatically, Ken brought the question to me, and it was several days before I realized that the only thing different between the 2nd PSA reading and the 3rd was his greatly increased water intake. Ken had always drunk copious amounts of coffee each day, but only one glass of water, and that's with his dinner.

Ken's tumor appears to be defeated, and the cancer cells in his bone tissue appear to be retreating. Ken continues to drink 8 glasses of water each day.

You are welcome to use any of these documents in any way you wish.

Sincerely, C. B.

Dear Dr. B.,

First I want to thank you profusely for writing that book! I can relate to your struggles with the medical establishment as I have opted for alternative methods other than chemo, radiation & surgery and have had to endure what I call the Western medical gauntlet, which is yet another story.

I don't know you, but I'm proud of you! You're one of the real heroes!

Some background: In April of 1997 I was diagnosed with squamous cell carcinoma of the left tonsil, which metastasized into the lymph nodes of the neck by Stanford tumor board. I was told I was in the most dramatic way that I had a 15 to 30% chance of survival if I followed their recommendations. These were to have a radical neck dissection, which included removing of the 11th cranial nerve, part of the jaw, and a lot of tissue in my throat, then radiation and 16 weeks of chemo. If I failed to follow recommended procedures my life span was expected to be over within a short 5 weeks! No one would give me a straight answer on costs, but it was reluctantly and unofficially estimated at $350,000 before the chemo. (By the way, I had an excellent health policy, which almost became my death sentence.)

After thoroughly looking at the options, I bailed out on the surgery, chemo, and the radiation. I started an organic macrobiotic diet, got rid of the toxins in and around my house, cleaned up my lifestyle, used some herbs, chi-gong, and eventually hyperbaric oxygen, which was very effective.

In the last 4 & a half years, I had the cancer looking like it was in remission, but then after a couple of years I slowly fell off the diet. The cancer started up again with four new tumors. I stopped it on this second occasion with the same regimen for many months, but could not reverse it. A doctor convinced me to cut back on the salt and in a few months I developed 6 more tumors. Up until now, I've never had much pain, or have ever lost a day of work. 20 days ago it has taken a jumpstart. Tumors have definitely grown. They may be encroaching on the carotid artery and probably the main nerve sheath. Some necrotizing tissue appeared on the tonsil, covering it within 3 days, possibly some bone loss in the jaw, and the worst part of it, some excruciating stabbing nerve pain that's off the scale. My latest prognosis was that within days I'd be sucked into the system with overwhelming pain or that I would bleed to death any time.

I just read your 1992 edition of Your Body's Many Cries for Water and got a strong feeling this cancer is due to long-term dehydration. I have drunk very little water in the past. I was given OxyContin for pain as well as Percocet. I don't like feeling the drug stupor so I opted to try two glasses of water & a pinch of salt as your book suggested. Amazingly, the water is much more effective for this kind of core pain than the drugs! In only 12 days, there is a change coming on in the tumors. They appear to be shrinking slightly, in any case, softening and changing to smoother shapes. The pain is dramatically disappearing.

This may be too early to say, but the necrotizing tissue on the tonsil seems to be clearing up. Thanks to your book, I hope I've discovered this in time, that ordinary water may be the missing link. Won't that be a testament if I can cure this cancer with your WaterCure??? The race is on.

So far, I've let the pain dictate my water consumption once I've drunk a liter & a half. This has brought me to 3–4 liters a day. I am a 52-year-old scuba charter boat captain and in excellent shape, other than this pesky cancer.

Thank you
Respectfully, E. C.

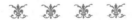

Dear Dr. B.,

In November 1988, I was diagnosed with bone marrow cancer and was told that my condition was terminal. For twelve years, I did not receive any type of chemotherapy.

Doctors do not understand how I can live so long with terminal cancer. Most patients with this type of cancer normally live three to six years, which was the life expectancy they gave me. They cannot understand why I do not have holes in my bones by now.

On August 4, 2000, I was taken to Parkway Medical Center's ER in the following condition:

1. Unconscious

2. Respiratory failure

3. Fever, temperature 104.8

4. Heartbeat was 222 beats per minute5. Blood pressure 200/130

6. Pneumonia

7. Bacterial meningitis (inflammation of the spinal cord and the lining of the brain)

8. Blood was sludge

9. Hemorrhaging from the nose

10. Multiple myeloma (bone cancer)

11. Zero immune system (due to bone cancer)

That same week it was reported on television that two healthy young men ages 17 and 21 died of meningitis. The doctors said that if I had arrived at the hospital two hours later I would have been dead upon arrival. Bacterial meningitis is the worst kind of meningitis a person can contract.

I was in ICU for ten days, unconscious and on a ventilator. The doctors did not think I was going to live. The primary-care physician informed my family that I might need a tracheotomy, having a feeding tube placed in my intestines, and be kept alive by machines. My family was informed that I might be a vegetable if and when I did wake up. The doctors said that most patients that have been unconscious and on the ventilator for the length of time I was, usually wake up brain dead.

By the grace of God, on the 11th day I woke up breathing on my own with all my faculties and a sound mind. Today, nine weeks later, I stand in God's amazing grace giving Him all the praise and all the glory. I am healed, walking in divine health. I am also still drinking a gallon and half of water with 1/2 tsp. of salt every day. Thanks to your teaching.

Sincerely, M. J.

BREAST CANCER

If ever a cancer story were to make you think twice about trusting the mainstream medical establishment and its offers of chemotherapy, radiation, and surgery, it is the firsthand experience of Lorraine Day, M.D., a renowned orthopedic surgeon herself, with many years of teaching hospital experience. For 15 years she was on the faculty of the University of California, San Francisco, School of Medicine—considered among the top three medical schools in America. She was an associate professor, vice chairman of the Department of Orthopedic Surgery, and chief of orthopedic surgery at San Francisco General Hospital itself, where she was involved in the training of thousands of doctors. She compares her daily routine when she was at S.F. General with the wartime field hospital portrayed in the TV series M*A*S*H.

Dr. Day was a frequent lecturer at many top medical institutions in America and Europe, including the Massachusetts Medical Society and the Royal Society of Medicine in London, England—both very prestigious centers of thought. In short, she was considered one of mainstream medicine's most highly qualified physicians, qualified enough to mold the minds of emerging doctors. At this point in her life, and at the peak of her dizzying medical achievements, the Creator enrolled her in His own medical school and threw her into the deep waters of the unknown, as He had with me a number of years before. She developed a very fast-growing breast cancer in 1992.

She immediately knew that what knowledge she had about cancer was not enough, and that the prevalent treatments she had used for her patients were not what she wanted for herself. As she correctly says, doctors are more afraid of cancer than other diseases. They know the treatments they offer others do not work.

Within days she realized she would die soon. Her initial small tumor, protruding through the middle of her chest from her left breast, grew to the size of a large orange in about three weeks. She could not rely on her medical colleagues at her own university to deal with her medical emergency. Based on her obvious sanity and the information she had gathered, she did not wish to be another victim of the commerce-protected cancer treatment protocol—she states, "I refused chemotherapy, radiation, and mutilating surgery because, as a medical doctor with years of experience, I saw thousands of cancer patients die, not from their cancer, but from the painful, maiming, destructive treatments we doctors give them!"

She stopped practicing medicine and became a student of "alternative medicine." She started reading copiously about the natural treatment procedures offered by alternative medicine practitioners. She changed her lifestyle and started to look into nutrition for answers to her problem. The cancer was growing and would soon begin to break her skin and ulcerate, exposing her to the additional problems of becoming infected. She found a surgeon to only remove the external tumor and did nothing about its fast-growing secondaries in the glands in her armpit, in the space above her collarbone, in her nose, and elsewhere—no chemotherapy and no radiation.

The cancer came back with a vengeance and grew at rapid rates all over again despite her new diet. She became so weak that she could hardly walk and was nursed in her bed. At these final stages of her life, when the archangel was getting ready to accompany her to the Pearly Gates—and she knew it, too—as if God wanted to make an ignorance-shattering point in medicine and set her up as another of His medical messengers, someone gave her a copy of my book *Your Body's Many Cries for Water*. All at once she realized the information in the book was speaking to her problem, and she began to drink water as if there were no tomorrow.

She realized the coffee she'd been drinking all those years between operations, in place of water her body wanted, had done the damage and set her up for the development of the cancer she was now facing. Below are some artistic renditions of the size and location of Dr. Day's cancer and its secondaries.

I asked an artist friend of mine, Lourdes Saenz, to produce these renditions of the tumor photos that Dr. Day has posted on her Web site, www.drday.com. I chose to use art instead of photos to encourage you to go to her Web site and acquaint yourself with the crusade she is now engaged in against the very mainstream medical establishment she represented as a shining star for so many years. The addition of water to Dr. Day's daily diet gave the archangel his

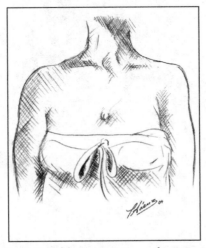

Art 1. Marble size tumor at the onset.

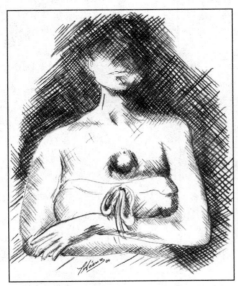

Art 1. Marble size tumor at the onset.

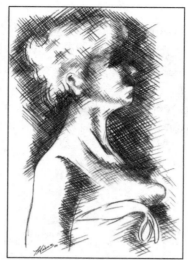

Art 3. This is the actual tumor and not the breast;
this growth occured in 3 weeks.

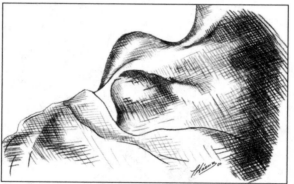

Art 4. Side view of tumor, extending deep into the tissues underneath.

marching orders, and she started feeling better every day. It took her about eight months to recover completely and become cancer-free—hallelujah. She has been cancer-free for the past ten years.

She now speaks at different conferences for the public, as well as to those from the medical establishment who are exercising intelligence and do not wish to hurt people now that a simpler alternative treatment protocol for cancer is available. Medical professionals whose family members develop cancer, or who have it themselves, seek her newly gained wisdom. She has adopted my book *Your Body's Many Cries for Water* as one of her teaching tools.

In March 2003 we met for the first time at a medical conference in Phoenix, Arizona. I asked her what made her think water played a pivotal role in the treatment of her cancer, when she is expanding her recommendations to include many different things. Her answer revealed the maturity of a true scientist. She told me she was doing all the other things before she incorporated water into her protocol, but without water they did not work. It was water that truly made the difference. Using all the other steps in her current recommendation, and no water, she was sinking fast and became immobile and was forced to stay mostly in bed. She has more than once stated:

"Dr. Batmanghelidj's book *Your Body's Many Cries for Water* was critical in my recovery. I could not have gotten well without that addition to my plan."

THE DEHYDRATION DRIVE OF BREAST CANCER

What could possibly speed cancer growth in the breast to the point that a tumor could expand to the size of a grapefruit, as in the case of Dr. Day? If I were to bet on any element in the chain of chemical events associated with dehydration, it would be increased prolactin production. Prolactin is one of the stress hormones of the body and also one of the hormones driving the gland tissue in the breast to produce milk.

Its increased production in stress is designed to compensate for the possible negative effect of dehydration on milk production. It is interesting to note that even birds have similar secretory glands in the back of their mouths, from which a kind of "milk" is squirted into the mouth of their chicks while in the nest. Milk, apart from being a source of energy and primary raw materials, also transfers the immunoglobulins of the mother to the child during the time that the child's immune system is not fully developed.

CHAPTER 7

STRESS HORMONES AND DEHYDRATION

Dehydration refers to the lack of free-to-use water needed to perform new metabolic functions in the chemical events that take place every second of every minute of every hour of every day of your life. Water that is not engaged in myriad other events and is free to break down proteins, starch, and fat actively drives the chemical events of the body into the immediate future. Your conscious mind may not recognize it, but having an inadequate water supply for a go-getter body is highly stressful and invokes a strong hormonal reaction that involves the secretion of vasopressin, endorphins, prolactin, and cortisone release factor, as well as the activation of the renin-angiotensin system.

These hormones further dehydrate the body because any available free water is used up to break down the stored raw materials and energy sources of the body to deal with continuation of the taxing business at hand. The body is mainly made up of water, but the bulk of that water is almost inaccessible to new undertakings. The "old water" you might have taken yesterday, or even a few hours ago, is already history. You need fresh intake of water to go forward into the future, without causing the body the stress of having to "to rob Peter to pay Paul," in which case the body becomes too concentrated and acidic—the very setup that initiates disease. Just as your car needs adequate gas for the trip you have planned, so your body needs sufficient free water in the blood circulation to make the journey of the day into the night, and beyond.

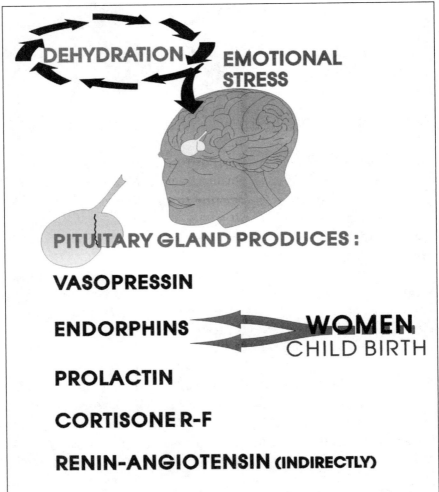

Figure 7-1. The stress-related hormones secreted by the pituitary gland.

Women, because of their traditionally stressing physiological events of monthly menstruation and childbearing, have a greater capacity for the production of two vital agents, endorphins and prolactin. Endorphins help them endure hardship more discreetly, and prolactin makes sure their offspring gets his or her water needs met in the form of milk, even at the expense of the mother herself. Of course the pituitary gland has many other hormones, such as the growth hormone, but these two have a great impact on the water regulation and metabolic mechanisms of the body when it is stressed.

We should look at milk as water that has other things to carry into the inner systems of a child. The composition of milk varies from species to species, depending on the growth cycle of the offspring. Cow's milk caters to the needs of a calf that walks within minutes of its birth. Cow's milk is more concentrated and has more fat than human milk. Human milk is more dilute—88.5 percent water, 3.3 percent fat, and 1.5 percent protein, while cow's milk is 87 percent water, 3.5 percent fat, and 4.1 percent proteins. Human milk is sweeter than cow's milk—6.8 percent lactose in human milk, compared with 4.8 percent in cow's milk.

Because of milk's very high water content—which is infinitely more important for an infant's survival than are milk's solids—the mother's breast is primarily a water fountain; the addition of other products to its water-manufacturing process is a secondary function.

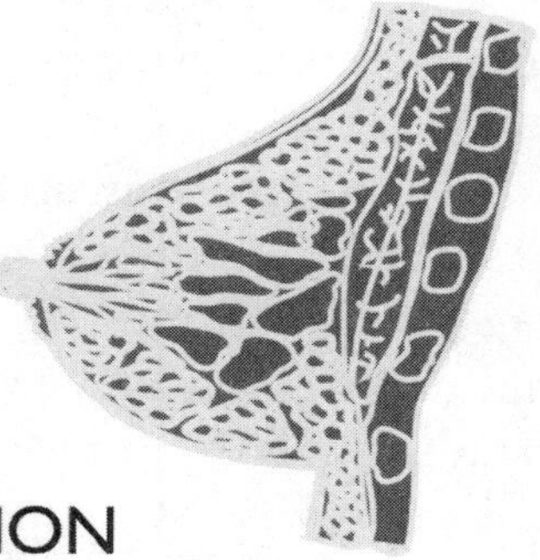

BREAST IS NATURE'S WATER FOUNTAIN TO A NEW BORN

PROLACTIN SECRETION INCREASED IN: DEHYDRATION, STRESS AND EXCESS DEHYDRATION, STRESS AND EXCESS ASPARTAME (DIET SODAS) INTAKE

EXCESS PROLACTIN SHOWN TO CAUSE

MAMMARY MICE

Figure 7-2. The elements that drive prolactin production in the body.

PROLACTIN AND DEPRESSION

Let me explain how the chemistry of depression at its onset can ultimately result in increased prolactin secretion and possible formation of cancer of the breast in women. Under normal conditions, all hormonal secretions have many checks and balances. Prolactin secretion in the body is a finely regulated process, until and unless outside factors negatively influence this fine regulation. I just explained its direct connection to stress.

However, its indirect connection is to the excess stress-induced destruction of the amino acid tyrosine and reduced production of dopamine. Dopamine is a neurotransmitter that prevents you from getting depressed. It strongly inhibits prolactin secretion. When brain dopamine levels fall off in depression, the drive for prolactin secretion continues unchecked, a catastrophic situation if the early stages of cancer cell development are present.

The artificial sweetener aspartame, used in more than 5,000 food products, is a major driver of prolactin secretion in the body. Aspartame breaks up into the amino acids aspartate, phenylalanine, and methyl alcohol. Methyl alcohol is a very strong nerve poison and is being blamed for many eye problems, such as macular degeneration. Phenylalanine is a bona fide amino acid the body can use, but aspartate is something to be concerned about. Aspartate traverses the blood barriers of the brain and directly influences the brain parts that deal with the reproductive organs. The breast is one of these organs. This is how seemingly innocuous aspartame intake can drive prolactin production in the body.

You now have some idea of how the immune-suppressive effects of dehydration can cause cancer in the body. I hope you better understand the cancer-preventive effects of proper hydration of the body, and also how some cancers can be reversed.

ANIMALS AND THEIR SALT CURE

An indispensable component of the WaterCure is a simultaneous adjustment of daily salt intake—unrefined salt that also contains the other 80 or more additional minerals found in the ocean. It is now clear that this kind of salt is also good for animals—in fact, very good for them. Good enough to cure some of their health problems. Below is the story of how it was discovered that salt should be added to the food of your pets.

Dr. Gary Weissberger is a practicing chiropractor in the area of Wilkes-Barre, Pennsylvania. He himself had a very bad pain in his foot that was not responding to treatment. He happened to run into Bob Butts—the person who has spent more than $400,000 educating the people of northeastern Pennsylvania about the WaterCure and the importance of salt for the relief of joint pains. Bob advised him to take some sea salt before going to bed. The result was the unexpected miracle of pain relief. Dr. Weissberger is now incorporating the WaterCure protocol into his practice. Here is his letter. I thought you might enjoy reading the views of a person who is engaged in the treatment of others, before we get into the discussion about cats and dogs.

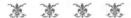

Dr. B.,

I would be most honored to have you include my story in your upcoming book.

The results that my patients are experiencing are wonderful now that they are following the WaterCure, but even more important to me personally is the lifelong friendships that are being forged, just because I am doing what is right.

Recently a patient started care with me because she saw an ad that Bob had placed in the newspaper. She is a very obese patient who could not leave her apartment because of her deteriorated medical condition and the fact that she recently fell and fractured her radius. She was quite amazed when she called to discuss the WaterCure and I told her I make house calls for people in need. Three weeks after I placed her on the WaterCure, I was shocked and amazed to learn that Mary not only lost thirty pounds in that short period of time, but she also managed to leave her apartment on her own and drove herself to a dr.'s appointment.

When I thought it couldn't get much better than this, on my last visit to Mary's apartment she surprised me with the fact that she placed my entire family on her daily prayer list! Money can't buy what that has done for me. Thank you from the bottom of my heart.

If I can be of any further assistance, please feel free to contact me at anytime

Sincerely, Dr. Gary Weissberger

You have another firsthand report from a doctor that water can help you lose weight. This doctor initiated the use of salt for the cure of arthritis pain in dogs and cats, and through him, the use of salt in the treatment of cancers in the same animal species. Here is Bob Butts's report on this matter.

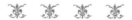

Dear Dr. B.,

It will be ten years in August since I met you, which was the start of the most exciting ten years in my life. While I have seen people cured of many incurable things, nothing has created more astonishment than the pets that are being quickly cured of terminal arthritis, most terminal cancers, and diabetes. The details of these stories are on my Web site, www.watercure2.com.

What started the animal cures was a salt skeptical chiropractor friend, Dr. Gary Weissberger, who still did not believe in the merits of salt even though he had found relief from his foot pain using salt a few years before. I decided that I was going to convince him and suggested that he try to find a person with a terminally ill pet with arthritis or cancer. Ask its owner to give the animal 1/2 tsp. of high-mineral sea salt in its quart dish with water and sprinkle a little sea salt on its food for three days and he'd be amazed.

Not having any experience with this on pets, but it made sense, especially when the only thing pets drink is water. That made it obvious that if pets and people both get arthritis and cancer, then the only other thing that could cause these problems in pets must be lack of good salt.

Two weeks later I get a call from Gary telling me he had a testimonial from Pete the dog. Pete, a dog that belonged to a naturopathic doctor, Dr. P. J. Marceletti of Tannersville, Pa., had terminal cancer and about a month to live. After three days on the salt, his tumor shrunk fifty percent. The astonished doctor then did the entire WaterCure on himself as he had an incurable problem called Crohn's disease. In a few days most of its symptoms vanished. That led to both doctors not only being convinced and prescribing the WaterCure to their patients. Both have done nonpaid TV spots here in northeastern Pa. telling of their exciting results.

Then there was a cat named Missy, belonging to Donna (afmprint@aol.com), who had breast cancer. They had taken her to Cornell University where the cancer was removed, but it came back. Donna read the articles that we had put in the major newspapers here in northeastern Pa. about pets getting rid of terminal diseases, so she tried the sea salt in her cat's food and water. In a short time Donna had a happy, healthy cat, which was back to jumping up on the bed & counters, racing up and down hallways, and keeping her dogs in line. Missy is not only back to her old self, she's even better. "I tell everyone about the WaterCure" were her comments.

A few days ago, president of the Luzerne County SPCA, Lorraine Smith of Diamond Ave., Wilkes-Barre, Pa., called excitedly to tell me of the results she has been seeing with pets that had severe arthritis, including her own dog. In a few days her dog was also running up and down steps. Barry Farber, who has a syndicated radio talk show, heard about our success with pets and asked us to participate in his Sunday show and share the good news with other pet owners. Lorraine appeared with me on his talk show on Sunday, July 25, 2004. She told a national audience about her experiences using sea salt to cure disease in pets in her charge.

A prominent Forty-Fort, Pa., veterinarian is now telling his clients to put their pets on sea salt because of the great results he has been seeing also, as are a number of other vets in the area.

Whatever skepticism some people may have had regarding the WaterCure appears to be melting away in the light of the tremendous results it is having on pets. These pet miracles are touching the hearts of their owners everywhere.

Please e-mail us your pet story along with a picture to drb@water-cure.com for a soon to be announced book about curing the so-called incurable diseases in our unconditionally loving pets.

Bob Butts

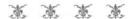

As you can see, there is more to salt as a medication than has been understood until now. Once again, the animal experience in medicine is coming to the aid of humans. Let us now get into the WaterCure treatment protocol for the treatment of cancer, obesity, and depression.

PART 4

THEIR NATURAL CURE

In this section, I have taken the liberty of repeating some of the information that's also provided here and there throughout this book. I am doing so to provide you with the total picture of the importance of water to health, well-being, disease prevention, and recovery from disease. I have assumed that you will benefit from reading information on dehydration more than once in order to master it. This section also offers more details on specific amounts of water, minerals, and food components to include in the treatment protocol for reversing obesity, depression, and cancer.

CHAPTER 8

THE IDEAL DIET FOR ALL
DEHYDRATION-PRODUCED DISEASES

Chronic dehydration produces many symptoms, signs, and eventually degenerative diseases. The physiological outcomes of the sort of dehydration that produces any of the problems mentioned earlier in the book are almost the same. Different bodies manifest the early symptoms of drought differently, but in persistent dehydration that has been camouflaged by prescription medications, one by one the other symptoms and signs will kick in, and eventually the person will suffer from multiple "diseases."

You saw it in the case of Andrew Bauman. We in medicine have labeled these conditions as outright diseases or have grouped them as different "syndromes." In recent years, we have grouped some of the syndromes—with some typical blood tests—and called them autoimmune diseases, such as lupus, multiple sclerosis, muscular dystrophy, insulin-dependent diabetes, and so on.

Medical research has until now been conducted on the assumption that many conditions—which I consider to be states of dehydration or its complications—are diseases of "unknown etiology." From the presently held perspectives of human health problems, we are not allowed to use the word cure. You can at best "treat" a problem and hope it goes "into remission."

From my perspective, most painful degenerative diseases are states of local or regional drought—with varying patterns. It naturally follows that, once the drought and its metabolic complications are corrected, the problem will be cured if the dehydration damage is not extensive. I also believe that to evaluate "deficiency disorders"—water deficiency being one of them—we do not need to observe the same research protocols that are applied to the research of chemical products. Identifying the shortage and correcting the deficiency are all we need do to cure the problem. Deficiency disorders are curable; we can use the word cure to refer to the result!

It is now clear that the treatment for all dehydration-produced conditions is the same—a single treatment protocol for umpteen numbers of conditions. Isn't that great? One program solves so many problems and avoids costly and unnecessary interference with the body.

The first step in this treatment program involves a clear and determined upward adjustment of daily water intake. Persistent dehydration also causes a disproportionate loss of certain elements that should be adequately available in the stored reserves in the body. Naturally, the ideal treatment protocol will also involve an appropriate correction of associated metabolic disturbances. In short, treatment of dehydration-produced diseases also involves correction of the secondary deficiencies that water deficiency imposes on some tissues of the body. This multiple-deficiency phenomenon caused by dehydration is at the root of many degenerative diseases, including the autoimmune conditions like lupus and AIDS and, naturally, cancer.

HOW MUCH WATER AND WHEN?

The body needs no less than two quarts of water and some salt every day to compensate for its natural losses in urine, respiration, and perspiration. Less than this will cause a burden on the kidneys, which will have to work harder to concentrate the urine, excreting as much chemical toxic waste in as little water as possible. This process explains why so many people end up needing dialysis in the final years of their drastically shortened lives.

By and large, an average-sized body needs about four quarts of water a day. You give it two quarts in form of water; the other two quarts are supplied from metabolism and the water content of food. The body needs these four quarts of water to produce around two quarts of urine—an amount that will prevent your kidneys from working too hard to concentrate the urine (thus the light-colored urine of well-hydrated people). Your lungs use more than a quart of water a day—this much water is evaporated in the process of breathing. The rest of the water is needed for perspiration and proper hydration of the skin, which is constantly losing water into the air around it. Some water is also needed for keeping feces moist to facilitate bowel movements. In hot climates more water is needed for this purpose.

A rough rule of thumb for those who are heavyset is to drink 1/2 ounce of water for every pound of body weight per day. A 200-pound person thus needs 100 ounces of water daily.

Water should be taken anytime you're thirsty, even in the middle of a meal. Water intake in the middle of a meal does not drastically affect the process of digestion, but dehydration during food intake does.

Drink at least two glasses of water first thing in the morning to compensate for the water loss during eight hours of sleep. Here are the best times to take water during the rest of the day.

Half an hour before each major meal of the day, drink one or two glasses of water and give it time to establish its regulatory processes before you introduce food into your system. Those suffering from obesity, depression, or cancer should make sure to drink two glasses. During that half hour, the water is absorbed into the system and is once again secreted into the stomach, preparing it to receive solid foods. When you drink water before food, you avoid many problems of the gastrointestinal tract, including bloating, heartburn, colitis, constipation, diverticulitis, Crohn's disease, hiatal hernia, cancers of intestinal tract, and of course weight gain.

Two to two and a half hours after you've eaten, drink another 8–12 ounces of water (depending on the amount of food consumed). This will stimulate the satiety hormones and wrap up the digestive processes in the intestinal tract. It will also keep you from experiencing a false sensation of hunger when your body is simply craving more water to complete the digestion of already eaten food.

Water should be taken at regular intervals throughout the day to avoid thirst. Be sure to drink water before any physical activity, such as going for a walk or other more strenuous forms of exercise that cause sweating. I will explain how much salt to take later in this book.

CORRECTING THE COMPLICATIONS
OF DEHYDRATION

A change of lifestyle is vital for the correction of any dehydration-produced disorder. The backbone of the WaterCure program is:

- Sufficient water and salt intake.
- Regular exercise.
- A balanced, mineral-rich diet that includes lots of fruits and vegetables, and the fats needed to make cell membranes, hormones, and nerve insulation. Please abandon your cholesterol hang-up.
- Exclusion of caffeine and alcohol.
- Meditation to detoxify stressful thoughts.
- Exclusion of artificial sweeteners.

Also remember that the sort of dehydration that manifests itself in asthma leaves other scars within the body. This is why asthma in childhood is so devastating and can expose a child to so many health problems in later life, as you saw in the case of Andrew Bauman. My understanding of the damaging effects of dehydration during childhood is the reason I have been concentrating my efforts on eradicating asthma among children.

Why Is Water So Important for the Prevention and Cure of Obesity, Depression, and Cancer?

Here are the primary functions of water in the body:

- Water is the vehicle of transport for circulating blood cells—the core of the immune system.

- Water is a solvent for critical materials, including oxygen and the minerals that maintain the body cells in their plum-like state.

- Water is the bulk material that fills empty spaces in the body.

- Water is the adhesive that binds solid parts of the cell together by forming a membrane or protective barrier around the cell. In dehydration, this adhesive responsibility is passed on to cholesterol.

- The neurotransmission systems of the brain and nerves depend on rapid movement of sodium and potassium in and out of the membranes along the full length of the nerves. Water that is loose and not bonded with something else is free to move across the cell membrane and turn the "element-moving" pumps.

- Some of the element-moving pumps are voltage-generating pumps. Thus, efficiency of neurotransmission systems depends on the availability of free and unengaged water in nerve tissues. In its osmotic urge to get into the cell, water generates energy by turning the pump units that force potassium into the cell and push sodium outside the cell—much like water turning the turbines at a hydroelectric dam to make electricity.

- A cell membrane has two layers; between these layers is a constantly moving canal of water in which most outside messages are processed. In dehydration, the enzyme activity in this canal becomes less efficient, and the cell becomes correspondingly less active in its natural functions. This is when cholesterol gets used in the cell membrane to prevent further dehydration, figure 8-1.

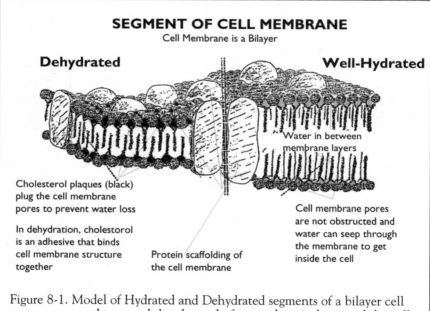

Figure 8-1. Model of Hydrated and Dehydrated segments of a bilayer cell membrane and the channel of water that circles round the cell in between the two layers of the membrane. The channel acts as a "water highway," where all the chemical exchanges of the cell with its outside world is carried out.

- Up to now, however, it has been assumed that all energy storage in ATP (adenosine triphosphate)æthe substance that "burns" and gives out "heat" to "cook" any of the chemical reactions allowing a cell to functionæis from food intake. This is why water has not received much attention as a source of energy in the energy-generating systems in the body.

- Water is the central regulator of energy and osmotic balance in the body. Sodium and potassium stick to the protein of the pump and act as the magnets of the dynamo. When water rotates the pump proteins, electricity is generated. The rapid turn of these cation pumps generates energy that is stored at many different locations in three different pool types:

  1. ATP is one type of energy pool.

  2. Another energy storage pool is GTP (guanosine triphosphate).

  3. A third system is in the endoplasmic reticulum that captures and traps calcium. For every two units of calcium that are trapped, the energy equivalent of one unit of ATP is stored in the connection of the two calcium atoms. For every two units of calcium that are separated from one another and released, one unit of energy—to make a new unit of ATP—is also released. This mechanism of calcium entrapment, as a means of energy storage, makes the bone structure of the body not only its scaffolding but also its "Fort Knox"—sort of like investing your cash in gold reserve. Hence, when there is severe dehydration and, consequently, a decreased supply of hydroelectric energy, the body taps into the bones for their energy storage. Thus, the primary cause of osteoporosis is persistent dehydration.

To prevent osteoporosis, or soft bones, you need to increase bone density by making the absorption of calcium more efficient. Toward this end, more vitamin D has to be made from solar conversion of cholesterol deposits in the skin to cholecalciferol—vitamin D3.

Cholesterol is the building block for practically all hormones of the body; vitamin D is also produced from cholesterol. This connection of high turnover of stored energy in the bone structure to an increased need for vitamin D activity to rebuild the bones is the signal for the liver to make more cholesterol as the precursor to vitamin D. It is a marker of scientific ignorance to attempt to lower choles-

terol levels via chemicals. Increased water intake and exposure to some sunlight is a less harmful way to regulate cholesterol levels of the circulating blood.

Cholesterol-lowering medications are dangerous. I have
mentioned some of their problems earlier in the book. Here
is another eye-opener for you. Duane Graveline, M.D.—a
former NASA astronaut, USAF flight surgeon, and space
medicine research scientist—published an article in the
August–September 2004 issue of the Townsend Letter for
Doctors and Patients called "Transient Global Amnesia: A
Side Effect of Statin Treatment." Dr. Graveline's own devastating experience led him to research this problem.

He has identified complete memory loss as one of the side
effects of cholesterol-lowering medications. He states: ". . .
thousands of case reports of memory dysfunction started
flooding in from patients across the country, all with the
same common thread—association with statin drug use.
And the amnesia is just the tip of the iceberg of the true
incidence of memory impairment associated with Lipitor,
Mevacor, and Zocor. For every case of amnesia, thousands
of cases of extreme forgetfulness, incapacitating confusion
and profound disorientation have been and are being
reported. Neither patients nor doctors are aware of this side
effect."

- The foods that we eat are the products of energy conversion
  from the initial electrical-energy-generating properties of
  water and sunlight. All living and growing species, humans
  included, survive as a result of energy generation from water.
  One major problem in the scientific evaluation of the body is
  the lack of understanding of the magnitude of our body's
  dependence on hydroelectricity for energy.

- The electricity produced at the cell membrane also forces
  nearby proteins to align their receptive points and prepare for
  chemical reactions.

WATER IS THE FIRST NUTRIENT THE BODY NEEDS

Here are some of the other reasons why your body needs water every day:

- Without water nothing lives.

- Comparative shortage of water suppresses and eventually kills some aspects of the body.

- Water is the main source of energy—the "cash flow" of the body.

- Water generates electrical and magnetic energy inside each and every cell of the body—it provides the power to live.

- Water prevents DNA damage and makes its repair mechanisms more efficient—less abnormal DNA is made.

- Water increases greatly the efficiency of the immune system in the bone marrow where the immune system is formed (all its mechanisms)—including its efficiency against cancer.

- Water is the main solvent for all foods, vitamins, and minerals. It is used in the breakdown of food into smaller particles and their eventual metabolism and assimilation.

- Water energizes food, and food particles are then able to supply the body with this energy during digestion. This is why food without water has absolutely no energy value for the body.

- Water increases the rate of absorption into the body of essential substances in food.

- Water is used to transport all substances inside the body.

- Water increases the efficiency of red blood cells in collecting oxygen in the lungs.

- When water reaches a cell, it brings the cell oxygen and takes the waste gases to the lungs for disposal.

- Water clears toxic waste from different parts of the body and takes it to the liver and kidneys for disposal.

- Water is the main lubricant in the joint spaces and prevents arthritis and back pain.

- Water is used in the spinal discs to make them "shock-absorbing water cushions."

- Water is the best lubricating laxative and prevents constipation.

- Water prevents heart attacks and strokes.

- Water prevents clogging of arteries in the heart and the brain.

- Water is essential for the body's cooling (sweat) and heating (electrical) systems.

- Water gives us power and electrical energy for all brain functions, particularly thinking.

- Water is directly needed for the efficient manufacture of all neurotransmitters, including serotonin.

- Water is directly needed for the production of all hormones made by the brain, including melatonin.

- Water prevents attention deficit disorder in children and adults.

- Water increases efficiency at work; it expands your attention span.

- Water is a better pick-me-up than any other beverage in the world—and it has no side effects.

- Water prevents stress, anxiety, and depression.

- Water restores normal sleep rhythms.

- Water prevents fatigue—it gives the energy of youth.

- Water makes the skin smooth and prevents aging.

- Water gives luster and shine to the eyes.

- Water prevents glaucoma.

- Water normalizes the blood-manufacturing systems in the bone marrow—it helps prevent leukemia and lymphoma.

- Water is absolutely vital for making the immune system more efficient in different regions to fight infections and cancer cells where they are formed.

- Water dilutes the blood and prevents it from clotting during circulation.

- Water decreases premenstrual pains and hot flashes.

- Water and heartbeats create the dilution and "waves" that keep things from "sedimenting" in the bloodstream.

- The human body has no water storage to draw on during dehydration. This is why you must drink regularly and throughout the day.

- Dehydration prevents sex hormone production—one of the primary causes of impotence and loss of libido.

- Drinking water separates the sensations of thirst and hunger.

- To lose weight, water is the best way to go—drink water on time and lose weight without much dieting. Also, you will not eat excessively when you are only thirsty for water.

- Dehydration causes deposits of toxic sediments in the tissue spaces, fat stores, joints, kidneys, liver, brain, and skin. Water will clear these deposits.

- Water takes away the morning sickness of pregnancy.

- Water integrates mind and body functions. It increases the ability to realize goals and purpose.

- Water prevents the loss of memory as we age. It prevents Alzheimer's disease, multiple sclerosis, Parkinson's disease, and Lou Gehrig's disease.

- Water reverses addictive urges, including those for caffeine, alcohol, and some drugs.

BLOOD IS A RED RIVER OF WATER

Blood is normally about 94 percent water when the body is fully hydrated (red cells are actually "water bags" that contain the colored hemoglobin). Inside the cells of the body there should ideally be about 75 percent water. Because of this difference in water levels outside and inside the cells, an osmotic flow of water into the cells normally occurs. There are hundreds of thousands of voltage-generating pump units at the cell membranes, just like the turbines used in hydroelectric dams. The water that flows through them rotates these pumps. This rush of water creates hydroelectric energy. At the same time, and as part of the same process, elements such as sodium and potassium are exchanged.

Only water that is free and can move about—the water you drink—generates hydroelectric energy at the cell membrane. The previously supplied water that is now busy with other functions cannot leave its binding position to rush elsewhere. This is why water by itself should be considered the most suitable pick-me-up beverage and should be consumed at regular intervals during the day. The good thing about water as a source of energy is the fact that excess water is passed out of the body. It manufactures the needed energy to top up the reserves in the cells and then leaves the body with the toxic waste of the cells. It is not stored.

When there is dehydration because a person is not drinking enough water, the cells become depleted of their ready energy. They then habitually depend on more energy generation from the intake of food instead of water. In this situation, the body is pushed into storing fat and using its protein and starch reserves, because it is immediately easier to break these elements down than the stored fat. This is why 37 percent of the people in America are grossly overweight: Their bodies are engaged in perpetual crisis management of dehydration.

WATER IS THE PRIMARY SOURCE OF ENERGY

The word hydrolysis (loosening, dissolving, breaking, or splitting by the participating action of water) is used when water becomes involved in the metabolism of other materials. Activities that depend on hydrolysis include the breakdown of proteins into their component amino acids, and the breakdown of large fatty particles into smaller fatty acid units. Without water, hydrolysis cannot take place. It follows, then, that the hydrolytic function of water also constitutes the metabolism of water itself. What this means is that water itself needs to be broken down first—hydrolyzed—before the body can use the various components in food. This is why we need to supply the body with water before we eat solid foods.

Now that we are on this point, let me once again give you the figures that stress the importance of water as a supplier of energy, especially for brain functions.

$$MgATP^+ + H_2O = ADP^{3-} / ADPH^{2-} + Mg^{2+} / H+ + H_2PO^+ / HPO_4^{2-}$$
$$600 \qquad\quad 1500 \quad\; 600 \quad 998 \quad 1168 \quad 318 \quad 1251$$

Figure 8-2. Energy is measured in kilo Joules. One kilo Joule is the amount of energy required to raise the temperature of 1 pound of water 1 degree Fahrenheit.

One unit of magnesium-ATP from the stockpile of energy at the cell membrane has about 600 units of energy before it is hydrolyzed. When it is hydrolyzed into its component parts, the total energy content reaches to about 5,835 units. (These figures are taken from an article published by P. George and co-workers: Biochem Biophys Acta 223, no. 1, 1970.)

All the foods that we eat and digest need to be hydrolyzed before the body can tap into their contents. The benefits they offer the body become available because of the "magical" effect of water, which breaks the products into their more easily digestible and water-energized components.

Now you know why water is a nutrient and how it generates energy. Water dissolves all the minerals, proteins, starches, and other water-soluble components and, as blood, carries them around the body for distribution. Think of blood as seawater that has a few breeds of fish in it—red cells, white cells, platelets, proteins, and enzymes, all swimming to a destination. The blood serum has almost the same mineral consistency and proportions as seawater.

The human body is in constant need of water. It is losing water through the lungs when we breathe out. It is losing water in perspiration from the skin, in urine production, and in daily bowel movements. A good gauge for the water needs of the body is the color of urine. A well-hydrated person produces colorless urine—not counting the color of vitamins or color additives in food. A comparatively dehydrated person produces yellow urine. A truly dehydrated person produces urine that is orange in color. Also: A well hydrated person is never constipated; a constipated person is truly a dehydrated person!

In the pages that follow, the importance of minerals and food components are briefly discussed. For a more thorough understanding of the importance of nutrition in maintaining health and well-being, I recommend the following book. *A Complete Illustrated Guide to Vitamins and Minerals*: A Practical Approach to a Healthy Diet and Safe Supplementation by Denise Mortimore, BSe, PhD, DHD: ISBN 0607-2717-1. You will enjoy reading this book.

CHAPTER 9

MINERALS ARE VITAL

Certain minerals need to pass through the acidic environment of the stomach before they can be absorbed through the mucosa of the intestine. They are zinc, magnesium, manganese, selenium, iron, copper, chromium, and molybdenum. They are listed in the order, in my view, of each element's importance to the human body. The mineral elements that the body needs in largest quantities are sodium, potassium, calcium, and magnesium. All one-a-day vitamin supplements are now composed such that the daily requirements of the essential minerals—other than sodium, calcium, and potassium—are provided. The rest of the vital minerals are fully available in the variety of foods we eat. The reason vitamin and mineral supplements are recommended is for "insurance" in case the daily diet is not high quality and you don't eat enough fruits and vegetables.

The toxic mineral elements are mercury, lead, aluminum, arsenic, cadmium, and, in large quantities, iron. These minerals should be avoided—they are absorbed better by the body if the stomach is less acidic than normal.

As we grow older, some of us manufacture less and less acid in our stomachs, even none. The condition is called achlorhydria. People with achlorhydria can become deficient in vital minerals. They also have difficulty in digesting meat and solid proteins.

In older cultures, eating pickles with food is a precautionary measure to prevent this problem. The use of vinegar in salads eaten with meals has the same effect. If the meal contains a lot of meat, the stomach normally secretes plenty of acid to break down the meat into small digestible particles, which are then further reduced to the size of their amino acid components before they pass into the intestines and get absorbed. People who have difficulty digesting food should get into the habit of taking some lemon or pickles with their food.

WHY WE HAVE MINERALS IN THE BODY

Next to water, minerals are the backbone of cell physiology. Although they are represented in the blood to a lesser extent, potassium, calcium, magnesium, zinc, selenium, chromium, copper, manganese, boron, vanadium, silicon, and some others maintain life inside the cells of the body. There are more of them inside the cells than there are in the blood. The first thing they do is osmotically hold on to water and regulate the plum-like volume and structure of the cells from inside. They also regulate the acid–alkaline balance inside the cell.

When these elements are adequately present in the cell interior, they osmotically and naturally pull and keep water in the cell. When these elements are less than adequately available, the method of water delivery into the cells is by forced injection through "showerheads," which are formed in the cell membrane to let only water in (figure 6-6). To do this, added pressure—injection pressure—is needed.

Proportionate to the level of mineral deficiency in the cell interior, injection pressure is adjusted to do the work. At a certain level, the rise in injection pressure becomes significant and is called hypertension. Hypertension denotes mineral deficiency in the interior of the cells of the body—a state of general mineral deficiency. Once this deficiency is corrected, and in conjunction with adequate salt intake, the blood pressure becomes normal once again. The more functionally important intracellular minerals are: Potasium, Calcium, Magnesium, Zinc and Selinium.

THE FUNCTIONAL SIGNIFICANCE OF SOME ESSENTIAL MINERALS

POTASSIUM is the primary water regulator of the cell interior. When it gets into the cell it osmotically holds onto the water that follows it into the cell. The plum-like state of a well-hydrated cell depends on the adequate presence of potassium within the cell. It osmotically balances the volume of water within the cell with the osmotic force of the environment outside the cell. Sodium is responsible for the osmotic force exerted by the extracellular fluid environment. Ultra fast pumps constantly regulate the mineral distribution inside and outside the cells. One such pump works with sodium and potassium exchange. They push 2 potassium atoms into the cell and in exchange pull 3 sodium atoms out of the cell.

The work of these pumps is responsible for the "osmotic push and pull of life."

Potassium has a tendency to leak to the exterior of the cell and has to be constantly pushed back. In dehydration, the energy to push the potassium back into the cell may be inadequate and some of this potassium may be lost to the body by its excretion in the urine. A great amount of potassium is also lost in heavy sweating. The loss of potassium from the cell will result in intracellular water loss—dehydration that will become chronic unless more water and some high potassium-containing foods are added to the daily diet. Continued pattern of potassium loss from the body will result in excess sodium retention by the kidneys and the first stages of high blood pressure, raised cholesterol, heart disease and irregular pulse will ensue.

The foods that have high potassium content are dried fruits like raisins, dried plums, dried apricot and dates. Potatoes, avocado, broad-, lima- and mung beans are also high in potassium. Banana, tomato, cauliflower, whole-wheat bread, peas, orange, milk, yogurt, eggs and cheese are also fairly rich in potassium.

If you are concerned with high blood pressure and heart disease, make sure your diet contains much more of the intracellular minerals than you take sodium. An adult needs up to 4 grams of potassium in his diet. A balanced diet is the best way to get one's minerals. Do not take too much orange juice just because it is high in potassium. You can add carrot juice and tomato juice and vegetable juice to your daily diet. They are high in potassium too.

CALCIUM and magnesium are electrogenic minerals. Their movement into the cell generates voltage, in the same way that sodium and potassium are said to manufacture electricity. This electrical current is used up to "cook" chemical reactions. Naturally, these elements produce voltage if water is around to dictate their relocation by the special proteins that act as mineral-specific pumps.

Calcium is the most abundant mineral in the body. It traps energy and holds on to it in the bone structure until the energy has to be released and calcium atoms are either recycled or passed in the urine. Release of energy from its calcium source is a kind of last-resort process. This is when bones become soft and lose their density, to the point that they are a constant source of pain when you put pressure on them. The run on stored energy in bone calcium and osteoporosis begin when the body gets persistently dehydrated and cannot manufacture sufficient hydroelectric energy.

In this physiological impasse, when the body is not producing sufficient urine because of dehydration, the excess calcium released from its bone deposits will obstruct the fine ducts in the kidneys; eventually, renal stones are formed that will ultimately destroy the renal organs. At some point, such patients will have to be dialyzed to stay alive for a few more months, or possibly years. Some get renal transplants. But had they taken the precaution of drinking water on a regular daily basis, they would have saved their kidneys and not have to face such dire options.

All the glands that secrete their hormones or manufacture enzymes for different digestive actions depend on the action of calcium before they can release their products.

Foods rich in calcium include milk and its by-products, such as cheese and yogurt; seeds like sesame and pumpkin; beans, figs, pulses, watercress, different nuts, olives, broccoli, dried fruits, eggs, potatoes, and all the green leafy vegetables.

MAGNESIUM is the element that gives stability to all energy-dependent processes in the brain, heart, kidneys, liver, pancreas, reproductive organs, and more. It is the affinity of magnesium-ATP for water that expands its energy content by almost one order of magnitude—600 units of energy become 5,835 when water breaks it down. When nine trillion brain and nerve cells communicate with one another, it is the reserves in magnesium energy pools that permit such activity. The heart muscle, which has to beat incessantly from its first moment of creation to the last moment of life, depends on the vital functions of magnesium for its contractile strength and rates of regular contraction. The formula given earlier for hydrolysis of magnesium-ATP shows how magnesium is used in the energy distribution in physiological function of cells, be they muscle cells, brain cells, or liver cells.

Of the minerals inside the cell, all are vitally important, but magnesium has a role that permits perpetuity of function, and the lack of it will impact a cell's efficiency and duration of its useful life. Magnesium is involved in more than 300 enzymatic reactions concerning protein, starch, and fat metabolism. Blood sugar regulation could benefit from additional availability of magnesium. Magnesium deficiency in the body is a very serious unrecognized problem.

Hard water is a good source of magnesium. People who drink hard water seem to be less prone to heart disease and irregular heartbeat. Low levels of magnesium in the diet will eventually be an additional cause of hypertension and irregular heartbeat—a major indicator of magnesium deficiency in the body. The diet should contain more magnesium than calcium, with the approximate ratio of 2.5:1. Magnesium in the natural water we drink can contribute to the daily needs of the body. People who have bought into the idea that distilled water or even drinking water after filtration through an RO system is good for them must bear in mind they will need to remineralize the water before drinking it.

Carbonated drinks and sodas contain much phosphate. Phosphate rids the body of magnesium. Weight for weight, phosphate will get rid of magnesium at a rate that equals the phosphate taken in. In short, the more phosphates you take in, the more magnesium-depleted you become. Sodas, other than the negative action of their caffeine content itself, are directly responsible for depleting magnesium from the body—a most perilous outcome and the likely cause of many unrecognized health problems associated with the intake of physiologically undesirable fluids.

Scientifically, it is now clear, "Aging is the direct result of multiple deficiencies in the body. It starts with dehydration followed by vital mineral deficiencies—with magnesium on top of the list." Everyone has to become aware of the importance of magnesium to well-being and efficient physiological functions. This includes the function of the immune system and recovery from serious diseases such as heart disease and cancers. It is safe to say that if you do not have a dehydration-produced mineral deficiency, you will not get sick. To recover from sickness, correct the dehydration and replace the lost minerals from your body.

Mineral replacement should include all minerals. Nature has seen to it that all of them are well represented in a balanced diet. Food is always a better source of these minerals. Unrefined salt is a "food." It contains more than 80 minerals, but its sodium content is more than your body could handle if you use it as your only source of the essential minerals it contains. The salt could be from the sea or from land deposits and mines. It should be in its natural state and composition—not stripped of its valuable combination of companion minerals.

Magnesium supply in foods is most abundant in the green of chlorophyll and in seeds—lentils, broad beans, peas, wheat bran, wheat germ, nuts such as almonds and peanuts, brown rice, barley, corn, and avocado. The highest level of magnesium in any plant is found in kelp, which is also rich in iodine. Milk and eggs also contain enough magnesium to make them wholesome foods.

ZINC is one of the most important minerals for accurate gene expression in the DNA assembly line. With the help of the amino acid cysteine, zinc holds on to some elements that are connected and bond to produce new enzymes and proteins. Don't forget that the internal environment where the DNA assembly line is positioned is watery; things could float away unless they are held in position until they connect. "Zinc clusters," "zinc twists," and "zinc fingers" are the various combinations of zinc structures that perform this highly specialized duty. Zinc is involved in the manufacture of more than 200 different enzymes and vital proteins in all the cells of the body. Now you see why zinc is not something you can afford to be without in your daily diet, particularly if you want to reverse a disease process like cancer. One protein that needs lots of zinc for its manufacture is the insulin receptor on the cell membranes—vital to correction of diabetic trends.

Popcorn is a very rich source of zinc. Most seeds like sesame and pumpkin are good sources as well. Beef, cheese, whole wheat, crabmeat, pecans, peanuts, lima beans, and peas are also good source of zinc; almonds, walnuts, eggs, and soybeans can contribute some zinc toward the daily needs of the body.

Alcohol, excess intake of calcium, excess intake of iron, low stomach acid (the most common cause after alcoholism), high dietary fiber intake, insufficient protein intake in the diet, and liver and pancreatic disease can contribute to zinc deficiency.

SELENIUM is similarly important to cell well-being. Shortages of selenium and zinc can wreak havoc on the normal functions of the body, particularly its immune system. Fortunately these elements are stored, and the body can tap into their reserves until cravings can steer you toward foods that are rich in these elements. Unfortunately, when the soil is depleted of these elements, they are not adequately represented in the local foods. It is said that the soil in East Africa is depleted of selenium, but the soil in West Africa is rich in it. One scientist has ventured the opinion that the reason for rampant spread of AIDS in East Africa, and not in West Africa, is the shortage of selenium in the local diet.

Selenium shortage can translate to lower levels of enzyme glutathione peroxidase seen in many forms of cancer.

Foods rich in selenium are wheat germ, different nuts, whole-wheat bread, brown rice, barley, beer, shrimp, oats, fish, mushrooms, garlic, and orange juice, and in lesser amounts pulses and cooked chicken.

SALT: THE ETERNAL MEDICATION

Salt is a vital substance for the survival of all living creatures, particularly humans, and especially people with asthma, allergies, and autoimmune disease.

Salt is a "medication" used by healers through the ages. In certain cultures, salt is worth its weight in gold and is, in fact, exchanged weight for weight for gold. In desert countries, people know that salt intake is their insurance for survival. To these people, salt mines are synonymous with gold mines. Salt has a biblical endorsement.

After many years of salt being bad-mouthed by ignorant health professionals and their media parrots, the importance of salt as a dietary supplement is once again being acknowledged and recognized. I was one of the early voices bringing about this change.

Water, salt, and potassium together regulate the water content of the body. Water regulates the water content of the interior of the cell by working its way into all the cells it reaches. It has to get there to cleanse and extract the toxic waste of cell metabolism. Once water gets into the cells, the potassium content of the cells holds on to it and keeps it there—to the extent that potassium is available inside the cells. Even in the plant kingdom, it is the potassium in fruit that gives it firmness by holding water in the interior of the fruit. Our daily food contains ample potassium from fruits and vegetables, but not salt from its natural source. That is why we need to add salt to our daily diet.

Salt forces some water to keep it company outside the cells (osmotic retention of water by salt). It balances the amount of water that is held outside the cells.

Basically, there are two oceans of water in the body: one held inside the cells and the other outside. Good health depends on a delicate balance between the volumes of these two oceans.

This balance is achieved by the regular intake of water, potassium-rich fruits and vegetables that also contain the vitamins that the body needs, and salt. Unrefined sea salt, which contains some of the other minerals that the body needs, is preferable.

When water is not available to get into the cells freely, it is filtered from the outside salty ocean and injected into the cells that are being overworked despite their water shortage. The design of our bodies is such that the extent of the ocean of water outside the cells is expanded to have the extra water available for filtration and emergency injection into vital cells. The brain commands an increase in salt and water retention by the kidneys. This directive of the brain is why we get edema when we don't drink enough water.

When water shortage in the body reaches a more critical level and delivery of water by its injection into the cells becomes the main route of supply to more and more cells, an associated rise in injection pressure becomes necessary. The significant rise in pressure needed to inject water into the cells becomes measurable and is labeled hypertension.

Initially, the process of water filtration and its delivery into the cells is more efficient at night when the body is horizontal. The collected water, which settles mostly in the legs during the day, does not have to fight the force of gravity to get into the blood circulation when the body is horizontal. If reliance on this process of emergency hydration of some cells continues for long, however, the lungs begin to get waterlogged and breathing becomes difficult. The person needs more pillows to sit upright to sleep.

This condition is called cardiac asthma and is the consequence of dehydration. However, in this condition you must not overload the system by drinking too much water at the beginning. Increases in water intake must be slow and spaced out—until urine production begins to increase at the same rate that you drink water.

When we drink enough water to pass clear urine, we also pass out a lot of the salt that was held back. This is how we can get rid of edema fluid from the body: by drinking more water. Not diuretics, but more water! Water is the best natural diuretic that exists.

In a person who has extensive edema and whose heart sometimes experiences irregular or very rapid beats with little effort, the increase in water intake should be gradual and spaced out, but water should not be withheld from the body. Salt intake should be limited for two or three days because the body is still in an overdrive mode to retain it. Once the edema has cleared up, salt should not be withheld from the body.

Salt: Some of Its Hidden Miracles

Salt has many functions other than just regulating the water content of the body. Here are some of its additional important functions in the body:

- Salt is a strong natural antihistamine. It can be used to relieve asthma: Put some on your tongue after drinking a glass or two of water. It is as effective as an inhaler, without the toxicity. You should drink one or two glasses of water before putting salt on the tongue.

- Salt is a strong anti-stress element for the body.

- Salt is vital for extracting excess acidity from inside the cells, particularly brain cells. If you don't want Alzheimer's disease, don't go salt-free, and don't let them put you on diuretic medications for long!

- Salt is vital for the kidneys to clear excess acidity, passing it into the urine. Without sufficient salt in the body, the body will become more and more acidic.

- Salt is essential in the treatment of emotional and affective disorders. Lithium is a salt substitute used in the treatment of depression. To prevent suffering from depression, make sure you take some salt.

- Salt is essential for preserving the serotonin and melatonin levels in the brain. When water and salt perform their natural antioxidant duties and clear toxic waste from the body, essential amino acids, such as tryptophan and tyrosine, will not be sacrificed as chemical antioxidants. In a well-hydrated body, tryptophan is spared and gets into the brain tissue, where it is used to manufacture serotonin, melatonin, indolamine, and tryptamine—essential antidepressant neurotransmitters.

- Salt, in my opinion, is vital for the prevention and treatment of cancer. Cancer cells are killed by oxygen; they are anaerobic organisms. They must live in a low-oxygen and acidic environment. When the body is well hydrated and salt expands the volume of blood circulation to reach all parts, the oxygen and the active and "motivated" immune cells in the blood reach the cancerous tissue and destroy it. As I explained, dehydration—shortage of water and salt—suppresses the immune system of the body and the activity of its disease-fighting immune cells.

- Salt is most effective in stabilizing irregular heartbeat, and—contrary to the misconception that it causes high blood pressure—it is actually essential for the regulation of blood pressure, in conjunction with water. Naturally, the proportions are critical. A low-salt diet with high water intake will, in some people, cause blood pressure to rise. The reason is simple. The essential intracellular minerals that are the natural components of unrefined salt are vital to keep blood pressure normal.

As a secondary complication, a low-salt diet can also cause asthma-like shortness of breath. If you drink water and do not take salt, the water will not stay in the blood circulation adequately to completely fill all the blood vessels. In some people, this will cause fainting, and in others, tightening of the arteries—and eventually constriction of bronchioles in the lungs—to the point of registering a rise in blood pressure, complicated by breathlessness. One or two glasses of water and some salt—a little of it on the tongue—will quickly and efficiently quiet a racing and thumping heart, and in the long run will reduce the blood pressure and cure breathlessness.

- Salt is vital for sleep regulation. It is a natural hypnotic. If you drink a full glass of water, then put a few grains of salt on your tongue and let it stay there, you will fall into a natural, deep sleep. Don't use salt on your tongue unless you also drink water. Repeated use of salt by itself might cause nosebleeds.

- Salt is a vitally needed element in the treatment of diabetics. It helps balance the sugar levels in the blood and reduces the need for insulin in those who have to inject the chemical to regulate their blood sugar levels. Water and salt reduce the extent of secondary damage associated with diabetes.

- Salt is vital for the generation of hydroelectric energy in all of the cells in the body. It is used for local power generation at the sites of energy needed by the cells.

- Salt is vital to the communication and information-processing of nerve cells the entire time that the brain cells work—from the moment of conception to death.

- Salt is vital for the absorption of food particles through the intestinal tract.

- Salt is vital for clearing the lungs of mucous plugs and sticky phlegm, particularly in asthma, emphysema, and cystic fibrosis sufferers. Salt makes mucus fluid and loose—ready to "disconnect"—by changing the physical state of its structure (the process is called charge-shielding).

- Salt on the tongue will stop persistent dry coughs; water will enhance this effect.

- Salt is vital for clearing up catarrh and sinus congestion.

- Salt is vital for the prevention of gout and gouty arthritis.

- Salt is essential for the prevention of muscle cramps.

- Salt is vital to preventing excess saliva production to the point that it flows out of the mouth during sleep. Needing to constantly mop up excess saliva indicates a salt shortage.

- Major osteoporosis is the result of salt and water shortages in the body. More than 20 percent of the salt reserves of the body are stored in the shaft of the long bones, giving them their strength. When the diet is short of salt, the stored salt in the bones is released to osmotically balance the content of salt in the blood. You can guess the rest.

- Salt is vital for maintaining self-confidence and a positive self-image—a serotonin- and melatonin-controlled "personality output."

- Salt is vital for maintaining sexuality and libido.

- Salt is vital for reducing a double chin. When the body is short of salt, it means the body really is short of water. The salivary glands sense the salt shortage and are obliged to produce more saliva to lubricate the act of chewing and swallowing and also to supply the stomach with the water it needs for breaking down foods. Circulation to the salivary glands increases, and the blood vessels become "leaky" in order to supply the glands with more water to manufacture saliva. This leakiness spills to areas beyond the glands themselves, causing increased bulk under the skin of the chin, the cheeks, and into the neck.

- Salt is vital for preventing varicose veins and spider veins on the legs and thighs.

- Sea salt and unrefined salt from salt mines contain about 80 mineral elements that the body needs. Some of these elements are needed in trace amounts. Unrefined sea salt is a better choice of salt than other refined salt on the market. Ordinary table salt bought in supermarkets has been stripped of its companion elements and contains additive elements to keep it powdery and porous. Aluminum is a very toxic element to the nervous system and until recently was used as an anti-caking agent in the preparation of table salt. Aluminum is implicated as one of the primary causes of Alzheimer's disease. If you see aluminum mentioned on the label of a salt container in the supermarket, don't buy it, and ask the manager to remove it from the shelf.

- Unrefined sea salt is now proving to be a pain and anticancer medication in animals—see the section on cancer.

- Salt is vital for maintaining muscle tone and strength. Involuntary leakage of urine could be a consequence of low salt intake that has resulted in the weakness of the bladder neck.

The following letter from Dottlee Reid, in her 60s, speaks volumes. It shows how salt intake helped her get over her constant problem of involuntary leakage of urine. I have chosen to print this letter here to share with millions of senior citizens in America the good news that adequate salt intake can possibly save them from the embarrassment of having to constantly wear pads.

Nov. 27, 1999

Dear Doctor Batmanghelidj:

June 25, 1999 I had to go home from work because the pain in my knee became unbearable. (This was an old wound, years ago caused by a chiropractor, that had been bruised again.) I was staying in bed a lot as it was too painful to try to walk.

Thank God Global Health Solutions got my name and address from somewhere and I got your book (Your Body's Many Cries for Water) and tapes. By July 3, 1999, I decided to try and walk around the block. I made it and July 4, 1999, I walked six blocks to church. On July 5, 1999, I rode seven hours only stopping twice to use the restroom. I have a very weak bladder and had even taken spare clothing, as I was sure they would be needed. I arrived with not a drop of anything on my clothing, and for the first time in my life I was not tired and I even took a walk before I went to bed.

I was very thin and was limited in what I could eat. Suddenly I find I am eating things I have not been able to eat in years—peaches, cantaloupe, watermelon, tomatoes, pineapple, and even sweets—and I was enjoying them with no side effects.

I had not been drinking anything but water for years, but I had talked myself off salt. A bad mistake! My muscles were really screaming as well as many parts of my body.

I still have problems to be worked out, but I'm learning how to listen to my own body and I hope to see the day I won't have any more problems with gas, digestion, circulation, and allergies. I can truthfully say most days I do feel better than I have in many years and I can never thank you enough for your help.

May God bless you as you try to help those He has placed on this earth.

Gratefully Yours Dottlee Reid

As much as salt is good for the body in asthma, excess potassium is bad for it. Too much orange juice, too many bananas, or any drink containing too much potassium might precipitate an asthma attack, particularly if taken before exercising—this can cause an exercise-induced asthma attack. To prevent such attacks, some salt intake before exercise will increase the lungs' capacity for air exchange. It will also decrease excess sweating.

It is a good policy to add some salt to orange juice to balance the actions of sodium and potassium in maintaining the required volume of water inside and outside the cells. In some cultures, salt is added to melon and other fruits to accentuate their sweetness. These fruits contain mostly potassium. By adding salt to them before eating, a balance between the intake of sodium and potassium results. The same should be done to other juices.

I received a call one day from one of the readers of my book to tell me how he had unwittingly hurt his son. Knowing that orange juice was full of vitamin C, he forced his son to drink several glasses of it every day. In the meantime, the young boy developed breathing problems and had a number of asthma attacks until he reached college and moved out of the sphere of influence of his father. His asthma cleared and his breathing became normal. The father told me he had to call his son and apologize for having given him such a hard time when he was younger. The more the son had rebelled against orange juice, the more the father had insisted he should take it, convinced a large amount was good for him.

How Much Salt?

As a rough rule of thumb, you need about 3 grams of salt—1/2 teaspoon—for every 8–10 glasses of water (depending on the volume of water in the glass), or 1/4 teaspoon per quart of water. You should take salt throughout the day. If you exercise and sweat, you need more salt. In hot climates, you need to take even more salt. In these climates, salt makes the difference between survival and better health and heat exhaustion and death.

When you get sick and land in the hospital, they immediately give you a saline IV drip with 0.9 percent concentration of salt. This figure translates to 9 grams of salt per liter of water. However, it is prudent to take a third as much salt on a regular daily basis—the body has a mechanism for preserving it.

Warning! You must at the same time not overdo salt. You must observe the ratio of salt and water needs of the body. You must always make sure you drink enough water to wash the excess salt out of your body. If your weight suddenly goes up in one day, you have taken too much salt. Hold back on salt intake for a day and drink plenty of water to increase your urine output and get rid of your swelling.

Those in heart failure—or kidney failure needing dialysis—must consult with their doctors before increasing their salt intake.

If you begin to drink water according to my protocol, you might also benefit from taking a one-a-day vitamin tablet daily, particularly if you do not exercise or eat hearty portions of vegetables and fruits. Meat and fish proteins are good sources of selenium and zinc. If you are under stress, and until it is over, you might consider adding some vitamin B6 and zinc to your diet in addition to what is available in the vitamin tablets.

If you suffer from cold sores (herpes simplex virus on the lips and even in the eyes) or genital herpes, make sure you add zinc and vitamin B6 to your diet. Your viral sores might very well be the result of zinc deficiency and its associated complications.

The true value of salt is in the added minerals it contains. Sodium is one of over 80 minerals contained in good salts. Table salt sold in supermarkets is stripped of its beneficial companion minerals and sold separately at much higher prices. Unrefined sea salt is now making its way into some supermarkets and health food stores. An even better source of salt is in the deposits that rare known as salt mines. Some come from Utah. Some are found in Mount Shasta. Salt from Himalaya is very popular in Europe and is now finding its way into America. These salt mines are many millions of years old and are less likely to have modern pollutants and impurities in them, unless they get used as the burial place of radioactive waste.

CHAPTER 10

PROTEINS

Experts are of the opinion that the body needs a minimum of between 1.1 and 1.4 grams of good-quality protein for every kilogram—2.2 pounds—of body weight per day. A 200-pound (90 kg) person needs about 4.5 ounces—120 grams—of protein a day to maintain his or her muscle mass. At this level of protein intake, the body will retain its normal composition of protein reserves and will not break into them and deplete some of the stored amino acids.

Children need a basic minimum of about 1 gram of protein for every pound of body weight.

In advanced societies that have high demands on their labor force for increased productivity, and have no food shortages, the recommended regular intake of protein seems to be around 10 ounces per day. The more physically active you are, the more protein-containing food your body needs. The extra protein is needed for tissue repairs and the manufacture of enzymes and neurotransmitters. High-protein diets are now fashionable in weight-loss programs.

Good-quality proteins can be found in eggs, milk, and legumes, such as lentils (which are 24 percent high-quality protein), mung beans, broad beans, soybeans, and tofu (extract of soybean). Vegetables also contain good-quality protein (spinach is about 13 percent protein), as do fresh turkey, chicken, veal, beef, pork, and fish. I use the word fresh because animal meat contains different enzymes that quickly destroy some of the essential amino acids within its proteins. Prolonged exposure to oxygen also destroys some of the essential amino acids in meat proteins. It makes the good fats in meat rancid and useless to the body. This is why in old cultures such as Chinese, Jewish, and Muslim, meat and fish have to be from a freshly killed source.

Do not take individual amino acids as supplements. At a certain concentration, some have adverse effects on the mineral and vitamin balance of the body. Amino acids in the body function more efficiently when they are proportionately represented.

EGGS

Eggs are a wholesome food. An average egg weighs 50 grams and has an energy value of 80 calories. The white of an egg weighs about 33 grams, and the yolk about 17 grams. One egg contains about 6 grams of top-quality proteins, no carbohydrates, and no fiber. The protein content of eggs is composed of a balanced range of amino acids. Eggs are rich in vitamins such as biotin, and minerals such as manganese, selenium, phosphorus, and copper. The yolk is a rich source of sulfur, a natural antioxidant that is now recognized as vital for health and well-being.

About 10 percent of an egg is its lipid or fat content. The lipid composition of the egg yolk is unique. It is rich in both lecithin, which is the precursor of the neurotransmitter acetylcholine, and DHA (docosa-hexa-enoic acid). DHA is an essential fat for maintaining brain function. It is needed for the constant repair of brain cell membranes and their cell-to-cell contact points—synaptosomes. The nerve structure of the eyes uses DHA for interpreting colors and for quality and sharpness of vision. Apart from being found in eggs, DHA is also found in cold-water fish and algae.

It is being increasingly understood that the level of cholesterol in the circulation is not affected by a high-egg diet. It is a medically published fact that an elderly man has for many years eaten about 24 eggs a day without any clinically significant rise in his cholesterol level.

There is no such thing as bad cholesterol! There are only uninformed and ignorant ideas that are exploited commercially to sell cholesterol-lowering drugs, which are actually more harmful to the body than slightly higher levels of circulating cholesterol.

The next time you come across a person who talks about "bad cholesterol" being the cause of heart disease, let that person know that we measure the level of cholesterol in the body from blood that is drawn from a vein. If it were true that higher levels of cholesterol cause plaques and obstruction of the blood vessels, then—because of the slower rate of blood flow in veins, which would encourage greater cholesterol deposits—we should also see much more blockage of the veins of the body. Since there is not a single scientific report of cholesterol deposits causing blockage of the veins, the assumption that cholesterol is bad and is the cause of heart disease is erroneous and unscientific. It is a commercial hype to sell expensive drugs and medical services. The sale of cholesterol-lowering drugs has leaped to $10 billion annually.

Let me once again explain why we get cholesterol deposits in the arteries of the heart or brain, or even on the inner wall of the major arteries of the body. Repeating my noncommercial scientific truth about cholesterol might better instill the information in your mind and save you from being conned. Remember, when I say dehydration I'm really referring to concentrated, acidic blood. Acidic blood that is also concentrated pulls water out of the cells lining the arterial walls. At the same time, the fast rush of blood against the delicate cells lining the inner wall of the arteries—weakened by the loss of their water and damaged by constant toxicity of concentrated blood—produces microscopic abrasions and tears.

Another of the many functions of cholesterol is its use as a "waterproof dressing" to cover damaged sites within the arterial membranes until they are repaired. Cholesterol acts as a kind of "grease gauze" that protects the wall of the artery from rupturing and peeling off and facilitates the easy flow of blood over its "greasy" surface. When you look at cholesterol from this perspective, you will realize what a blessing it really is; to blindly interfere with its physiological duties is irresponsible.

In my opinion, all the statistics about the level of cholesterol in the blood and the number of people who die of heart disease reflect the extent of the killer dehydration that has also caused the level of blood cholesterol to rise.

I will discuss another important role of cholesterol in the body later in this chapter. Based on my understanding of cholesterol, I have no hesitation in recommending eggs as a very good source of the essential dietary needs of the human body. I eat eggs almost every day. They are my preferred source of protein.

MILK PRODUCTS

For people who can digest milk products, natural, unsweetened yogurt is a good source of high-quality protein. It also contains lots of vitamins and good bacteria. The good bacteria in yogurt keep the intestinal tract healthy and help prevent the growth of toxic bacteria and toxic yeasts such as Candida. Of course, people who are allergic to dairy products should not take yogurt. Also make sure that the yogurt is not sweetened with aspartame—some brands are.

Cheeses are also a good source of protein. Freshly prepared cheeses are easier to digest and, in my opinion, are more wholesome than aged cheeses.

Some people cannot digest cow's milk easily. Although some contrary views about soy products are getting into print, until these views are verified beyond doubt, I still think soy milk is an acceptable substitute for cow's milk. After all, soy products have been for years the staple diet in China and other Asian countries—more than three billion people. If you do not like the taste of soy milk, mix it with carrot juice and enjoy the advantage of additional vitamins and nutrients. The combination is healthy and tasty. One drawback to soy in some people is its enlarging effects on the thyroid gland. These people may have to take extra iodine—contained in kelp.

FATS

Fat is an essential dietary requirement of the body. Some vital fatty acids that make up certain fats and oils are used as primary materials in the manufacture of cell membranes. They are also primary ingredients from which many of the hormones of the body are manufactured. The manufacture of sex hormones depends on the presence of some essential fats in the body, including the much-maligned cholesterol. Nerve cells need the "good" fats to remanufacture constantly used-up nerve endings.

The essential fat components are omega 6—a polyunsaturated fatty acid known as linoleic acid—and omega 3—a superunsaturated fatty acid known as alpha-linolenic acid. These fatty acids are in the form of oils.

Although some books claim that our bodies cannot make these essential fatty acids and have to import them in the form of oils in food, my recent discovery is the fact that the liver can indeed make these polyunsaturated fats. The following is a direct quote from page 756 of Guyton's Textbook of Medical Physiology, eighth edition: "Also, the liver cells are much more capable than other tissues of desaturating fatty acids so that the liver triglycerides normally are much more unsaturated than the triglycerides of the adipose tissue."

Naturally, these unsaturated fats get into the circulation and are distributed throughout the body to be used in the architecture of cell membranes. The brain is on top of the list of organs that constantly need unsaturated fats for the repair of membranes and nerve contact points.

All the same, a diet rich in polyunsaturated fats is most effective in certain other respects. One important effect of dietary unsaturated fats on the metabolism of the body is the moderate reduction in cholesterol formation by the liver, which produces practically all the cholesterol in the body—proper hydration has a similar impact on cholesterol levels of blood. I have mentioned these points to relieve the minds of the people, like myself, who are not disciplined enough to strictly stick to the "omega cult."

"Fat experts" say the average body needs between 6 and 9 grams of linoleic acid (omega 6) a day. It also needs around 2 to 9 grams of alpha-linolenic acid (omega 3), the most essential of the fatty acids. These fatty acids are needed particularly by the brain cells and their long nerves to manufacture insulated membranes, which need to be impermeable and prevent interference to the rate and flow of neurotransmission. The nerve endings in the retina involved in object recognition and clarity of sight have a high turnover of these essential fatty acids, particularly DHA. DHA is made from omega 3 fatty acid and is vital for brain cell composition. People with neurological disorders have been shown to be short of DHA.

As mentioned, eggs, cold-water fish, and algae are good sources of DHA. Another excellent source of the omega 3 and omega 6 fatty acids, in an ideal ratio of 3:1, is flaxseed (also known as linseed) oil that is cold-pressed and bottled in dark containers that keep out light. Light destroys these essential oils, which is why they are also packed in dark capsules. Sesame oil has the desirable property of being highly unsaturated. It is the eating oil of choice in many ancient cultures. Canola oil is also a good source of some essential fatty acids. The reason oils are better than solid fats is because at normal body temperature, they remain as oils and do not turn into sticky lard.

Butter is a rich source of fat-soluble vitamins, such as vitamin K, vitamin A, vitamin E, lecithin, folic acid, and more. Butter is also a rich source of calcium and phosphorous. The body needs some fat in its daily diet. You cannot go fat-free and survive for long.

The human body is basically a fat-burning machine. It prefers to convert starch and excess protein into fat and store it for use after it consumes its carbohydrate reserves. Glycogen is the form of carbohydrate that is stored in the liver and muscle tissue. The body has about half a day's reserve of glycogen. Before this reserve is depleted, the enzymes that burn fat are activated all over the body. In ideal situations, the protein is stored for repair works and the manufacture of enzymes and messenger chemicals. The fat is used for energy purposes and the manufacture of some hormones.

The only lifestyle action that will abort this naturally designed physiological process is repeated consumption of starchy foods or sweets that would stimulate the secretion of insulin. Insulin will stop the fat-burning enzymes dead in their tracks. This is how some people grow disproportionately fat. If you want to lose weight, your diet must contain some fat, preferably essential fatty acids, and fewer carbohydrates.

Each gram of fat provides the body with 9 calories of energy. Fat is a more efficient source of energy than starch, which has only 4 calories per gram. Our biological ancestors, who were basically hunter-gatherers chasing their food for long hours, could only do so because their bodies burned fat. More recently, our forebears became farmers with long days in the fields. They then graduated to pen-pushers in modern office settings with access to vending machines stocked with all kinds of taste bud stimulants, or with easy access to burger joints pushing french fries and starchy snacks—the cheapest forms of food.

Dr. Atkins understood this relationship of a high-fat and -protein diet to losing weight, but did not grasp the power of water in balancing the metabolic needs of the body. Most of his followers could not stick to their "waterless diet" and were not successful at maintaining their reduced weight. Some of his followers who also discovered the power of water are now the toast of Atkins chat room on the Internet.

FRUITS, VEGETABLES AND SUNLIGHT

The body needs fruits and green vegetables daily. They are ideal sources of the natural vitamins and minerals we need. Green vegetables also contain a great deal of beta-carotenes and even some DHA fatty acid, needed by the brain. Fruits and vegetables are important for maintaining the pH balance of the body. Chlorophyll contains a very high quantity of magnesium. Magnesium is to chlorophyll what iron is to hemoglobin in the blood—an oxygen carrier. In the human body, magnesium is the bonding anchor to the energy-storing unit within the cell membranes all over the body. The unit is called magnesium-adenosine-triphosphate (MgATP). If water reaches the MgATP pool and is enzymatically positioned to break it down, lots of energy will be released—this formula has already been presented.

SUNLIGHT: To asthmatics, sunlight is medicine. Light from the sun acts on the cholesterol deposits on the skin and converts them to vitamin D. Vitamin D encourages bone making and the entrapment of calcium by the bones—which in children helps them grow. Vitamin D also stimulates calcium absorption in the intestinal tract. Calcium has a direct acid-neutralizing effect in the body and is effective in balancing the cell pH—an outcome that alleviates asthma complications.

If you drink adequate amounts of water every day, take the required amount of salt, and get plenty of exercise—preferably in the open air and under good light—your body will begin to adjust its own intake of proteins and carbohydrates, as well as its requirements for fat to use as energy. Your need for proteins will increase. Your need for carbohydrates will decrease, and your fat-burning enzymes will consume more fat than is in the average diet. Contrary to the belief that cholesterol cannot be metabolized once it is deposited, it too will be cleared. The cholesterol deposits in your arteries may take longer to disappear than you might wish, but the body has all the chemical know-how to clear cholesterol plaques.

I repeat, there is no such thing as bad cholesterol. Remember that cholesterol is vital to physiology. We have to find out why the body sometimes manufactures more of it than usual.

When there is a shortage of water in the body, less hydroelectric energy is manufactured to energize all the dependent functions—like the low water flow in the river that feeds an electricity-generating dam. After a while, the dam will not hold enough water to operate all the generators. In real-life situations, when cheap energy from hydroelectric dams is insufficient, power generators begin to burn oil or coal to generate electricity.

In the body, the alternative source of energy is from calcium deposits in the bone or inside the cells. The energy trapped in the union of two fused-together calcium atoms is used instead. For each two calcium atoms bonded together, one unit of ATP energy is also trapped. The cells in the body have much trapped calcium in different storage sites; when these sites are broken up, their energy is used. There comes a time when this process results in the availability of too many loose calcium molecules—fuel ash. Fortunately, calcium ash is easily recycled. It needs vitamin D for its recycling process.

As I already mentioned, sunlight—energy—converts cholesterol in the skin to vitamin D. Vitamin D is responsible for facilitating the reentrapment of calcium and its reentry into the cells to be rebonded. Vitamin D sticks to its receptors on the cell membrane; simultaneously, one unit of calcium attaches itself to the exposed tail of the vitamin D in the process of entering the cell through the membrane. The union of calcium with vitamin D to the membrane receptor acts as a sort of magnetic rod—a whole chain of other essential elements and amino acids stick to the exposed calcium and are drawn into the cell.

In this way, the energy of sunlight and its conversion of cholesterol to vitamin D have direct physiological impact on the feeding of the cells of the body. When calcium reenters the cell, it takes other

essential elements with it. In this way, the cell receives raw materials for repair and energy metabolism. At the same time, the surplus energy that enters the cell is used to fuse together calcium
molecules and once again store energy in the calcium "bondage"
for future use.

Once you understand the logic behind the cascade of chemical
events in the body, you will realize the vital importance of cholesterol to cell metabolism and the health of the cells and bone structure. I need you to take a leap of faith with me and consider the
bones as a large reservoir of energy, which is stored in calcium
deposits. When the body is forced into breaking up calcium from
bones to tap into its stored energy, it is doing this well aware that
the bones become soft and less weight bearing—establishing osteoporosis. As a preventive measure, the level of cholesterol is raised
in the hope of having it "sun-energy-converted" into vitamin D to
start depositing calcium in the bones once again.

You should put the higher cholesterol levels of the body to full use.
Make more vitamin D from it and promote better-functioning and
fully utilized cells in your body. Use sunlight to your advantage to
lower your cholesterol.

Some of you might immediately react negatively to this statement
and express your fear of melanoma. It is my belief that cancers in
the body are produced by dehydration, inactivity, bad choices of
foods, and wrong beverages. For more than 20 years, I played three
hours of tennis six days a week in the heat of the early-afternoon
sun in Tehran. I did not develop any form of cancer. In support of
this statement, let me give you some information that was published in the Science Times of July 20, 2004.

Gina Kolata wrote about the views of Dr. A Bernard Ackerman, a
dermatologist with 625 research papers to his name. The good doctor, like me, does not believe sunlight is responsible for skin
melanomas, to the point that he went to Israel for a sunbathing
holiday and came back brown. He cites the obvious. Blacks and

Asians get their melanomas not on the parts of their bodies that are exposed to the sun, but on the areas that are unexposed, such as the soles of their feet, the palms of their hands, or even their mucous membranes. Whites develop melanomas mostly on their torsos and, in women, their legs—hardly exposed to the sun. Fair people, says Dr. Ackerman, should avoid exposing themselves to the sun for the sole purpose of preventing premature aging. You can take care of that concern by drinking more water.

You cannot sit at a desk in an artificially lit office and expect to have a normal cholesterol level. And in this situation, you will probably have a health professional who does not understand the mechanisms of sunlight energy conversion label this natural outcome of an incomplete chain of metabolic events a "disease," and a vital element, cholesterol, will be labeled as "bad."

I am certain this business of "bad cholesterol" is a slogan to fool people into using medications to lower it; by doing so, they get into harm's way so that someone else can get rich. Recently, an obviously commercially inspired "panel of experts" went even farther and lowered the safe level of cholesterol, to the point of commanding more people to take the appropriate drugs to avoid heart attacks. The charlatans know that if cholesterol does not block the veins in the body, it could not be held responsible for obstructing the arteries—there is not a single report of cholesterol ever having blocked a vein! Only God can save America from crooked professionals engaged in the business of medicine. They seem to be in charge in most places that matter.

EXERCISE

The most important factor for survival, after water, air, salt, and food, is exercise. Exercise is more important to the health of the individual than sex, entertainment, or anything else that might be pleasurable. The following points explain the importance of exercise for better health and a pain-free longer life.

- Exercise expands the vascular system in the muscle tissue and prevents hypertension.

- It opens the capillaries in the muscle tissue and, by lowering the resistance to blood flow in the arterial system, causes blood pressure to drop to normal.

- Exercise builds up muscle mass and prevents muscles from being broken down as fuel.

- Exercise stimulates the activity of fat-burning enzymes for manufacture of the constantly needed energy for muscle activity. When you train, you are in effect changing the source of energy for muscle activity. You convert the energy source from sugar that is in circulation to fat that is stored in the muscle itself.

- Exercise makes muscles burn as additional fuel some of the amino acids that would otherwise reach toxic levels in the body. In their greater-than-normal levels in the blood—usually reached in an unexercised body—certain branched-chain amino acids cause a drastic destruction and depletion of other vital amino acids. Some of these discarded essential amino acids are constantly needed by the brain to manufacture its neurotransmitters. Two of these essential amino acids are tryptophan and tyrosine. A more important role of tryptophan than its use as a precursor of neurotransmitters in the brain is its role in an enzyme system that recognizes and repairs incorrect DNA transcriptions.

The brain also uses tryptophan to make serotonin, melatonin, tryptamine, and indolamine, all of which are antidepressants and regulate sugar levels and blood pressure. Tyrosine is used for the manufacture of adrenalin, noradrenalin, and dopamine—vital for the coordination of body physiology when it has to take a physical action, such as fighting, running, playing sports, and so on. Excess tyrosine loss from the amino acid reserves of the body is also a primary factor in Parkinson's disease.

- Unexercised muscle gets broken down. As a result of the excretion of muscle parts from the body, some of the reserves of zinc and vitamin B6 also get lost. At a certain stage of this constant depletion of vitamin B6 and zinc, certain mental disorders and neurological complications occur. In effect, this happens in autoimmune diseases, including lupus and muscular dystrophy.

- Exercise makes the muscles hold more water in reserve and prevents increased concentration of blood, which would otherwise damage the lining of the blood vessel walls.

- Exercise lowers blood sugar in diabetics and decreases their need for insulin or tablet medications.

- Exercise compels the liver to manufacture sugar from the fat that it stores or the fat that is circulating within the blood.

- Exercise causes an increase in the mobility of the joints in the body. It causes the creation of an intermittent vacuum inside the joint cavities. The force of the vacuum causes suction of water into the cavity. Water in the joint cavity brings dissolved nutrients to the cells inside the cartilage. Increased water content of the cartilage also adds to its lubrication and smoother bone-on-bone gliding movements of the joint.

- Leg muscles act as secondary hearts. By their contractions and relaxations during the time we are upright, the leg muscles overcome the force of gravity. They pump into the venous system the blood that was sent to the legs. Because of the pressure breakers—and one-directional valves in the vein—the blood in the leg veins is pushed upward against gravity by frequent contraction of the leg muscles. This is how the leg muscles act as hearts for the venous system in the body. This is a value to exercise that not many people appreciate. Leg muscles also cause an equally effective flow within the lymphatic system and cause edema in the legs to disappear.

- Exercise strengthens the bones of the body and helps prevent osteoporosis.

- Exercise increases the production of all vital hormones, enhancing libido and heightening sexual performance.

- One hour of walking will cause the activation of fat-burning enzymes, which remain active for 12 hours. A morning and afternoon walk will keep these enzymes active around the clock and will cause clearance of cholesterol deposits in the arterial system.

- Exercise will enhance the activity of the adrenaline-operated sympathetic nerve system. Adrenaline will also reduce the over secretion of histamine and, as a result, will prevent asthma attacks and allergic reactions—provided the body is fully hydrated.

- Exercise will increase production of endorphins, enkephalins, and dynorphins, the natural opiates of the body. They produce the same "high" that drug addicts try to achieve through their abusive intake.

WHAT ARE THE BEST FORMS OF EXERCISE?

Exercising the body for endurance is better than exercising it for speed or for building excess muscle. In selecting an exercise, you should consider its lifetime value. A long-distance runner will enjoy the exercise value of long-distance runs into old age. A sprinter will not sprint for exercise at a later phase of life.

The best exercise that you can enjoy—even to a ripe old age, and without causing damage to the joints—is walking. Other exercises that will increase your endurance are swimming, golf, skiing, skating, climbing, tennis, squash, bicycling, tai chi, dancing, yoga, and aerobics. In selecting an exercise, evaluate its ability to keep the fat-burning enzymes active for longer durations. Outdoor forms of exercise are more beneficial for the body than indoor. The body becomes better connected to nature.

The four most vital steps to better health are: balancing the water and salt content of the body, exercising the muscle mass of the body—more effective in the open and in sunlight—taking a balanced daily diet of proteins and vegetables, and avoiding dehydrating beverages. These simple steps will be effective in prevention of the disease and are the foundation to any cure process the body needs to undergo.

FEREYDOON BATMANGHELIDJ, M.D.

Fereydoon Batmanghelidj, M.D., an internationally renowned researcher, author and advocate of the natural healing power of water, was born in Iran in 1931. He attended Fettes College in Scotland and was a graduate of St. Mary's Hospital Medical School of London University, where he studied under Sir Alexander Fleming, who shared the Nobel Prize for the discovery of penicillin.

Dr. Batmanghelidj practiced medicine in the United Kingdom before returning to Iran where he played a key role in the development of hospitals and medical centers. He also helped establish sport projects for youth in Iran, including The Ice Palace in Tehran, the first ice skating and sports complex in the Middle East.

When the Iranian Revolution broke out in 1979, Dr. Batmanghelidj was placed in the infamous Evin Prison as a political prisoner for two years and seven months. It was there he discovered the healing powers of water. One night, Dr. B. had to treat a fellow prisoner with crippling peptic ulcer pain. With no medications at his disposal, Dr. B. gave him two glasses of water. Within eight minutes, his pain disappeared. He was instructed to drink two glasses of water every three hours and became absolutely pain free for his four remaining months in the prison. Dr. B. successfully treated 3,000 fellow prisoners suffering from stress-induced peptic ulcer disease with water alone. While in prison he conducted extensive research into the medicinal effects of water in preventing and relieving many painful degenerative diseases. Evin proved an ideal "stress laboratory," and despite his being offered an earlier release, Dr. B. chose to stay an extra four months in prison to complete his research into the relationship of dehydration and bleeding peptic ulcer disease. The report of his findings was published as the editorial of the Journal of Clinical Gastroenterology in June 1983. The New York Times Science Watch reported this discovery on June 21, 1983.

On his release from prison in 1982, Dr. Batmanghelidj escaped from Iran and came to America. At the Foundation for the Simple in Medicine he began to research the effect of chronic unintentional dehydration on the human body. His findings were published in the Foundation's "Journal of Science in Medicine Simplified" in 1991 and 1992. They can be read on the web site www.watercure.com.

Dr. F. Batmanghelidj wrote his first self-help book "Your Body's Many Cries for Water" in 1992, in which he stated that a dry mouth is not a reliable indicator of dehydration. The body signals its water shortage by producing pain. Dehydration actually produces pain and many degenerative diseases, including asthma, arthritis, hypertension, angina, adult-onset diabetes, lupus and multiple sclerosis. Dr. B's message to the world is, "You are not sick, you are thirsty. Don't treat thirst with medication."

Dr. F. Batmanghelidj devoted the last 20 years of his life promoting public awareness of the healing powers of water. He appeared on hundreds of radio and television programs and lectured around the world. He has left a body of valuable works of six books and more than a dozen educational audio and video seminars. His work has created an international community that has embraced the natural healing of the water cure. His ground-breaking book "Your Body's Many Cries for Water" has been translated into 15 languages and continues to inspire readers all over the world.

Dr. F. Batmanghelidj died of complications from pneumonia on November 15, 2004, in Virginia, U.S.A. He was 73.

INDEX

OTHER HEALTH EDUCATION PRODUCTS
BY F. BATMANGHELIDJ, M.D.

BOOKS

YOUR BODY'S MANY CRIES FOR WATER
The Best-Selling Book
That has Brought Natural Healing to Millions!

This easy-to-read book is your guide to recognizing when your body is calling for water instead of costly prescription drugs (and their dangerous and life-threatening side effects). You'll get a better understanding of how unintentional dehydration is often the root cause of many painful degenerative diseases like asthma, allergies, hypertension, obesity and depression. Among other things, you will learn how to use water to eliminate pain, including heartburn, back pain, arthritis, angina and migraine headaches. Asthma can be cured in a few hours to a few days, naturally and forever. Also, lose weight effortlessly without denying yourself your favorite foods. Learn how to control your blood pressure and cholesterol levels naturally, and prevent sudden heart attacks.

ISBN: 0962994235
Paperback, 200 pages, $14.95
Packaging and postage, single book, $5.00

HOW TO DEAL WITH BACK PAIN AND RHEUMATOID JOINT PAIN

This educational, preventive-treatment manual gives you easy-to-use techniques for relieving chronic back pain and rheumatoid joint pain. It's the ideal accompaniment to Dr. Batmanghelidj's video, "How to Deal with Back Pain," since it illustrates and explains the easy-to-do corrective body movements for instant and lasting back pain relief. You will learn the importance of maintaining the proper alkalinity in your body's cells and how water and salt can be used to wash away the acidity that causes pain. You will understand the structure of your body's spinal column, vertebrae and joints – made easy with the book's clearly presented pictures, graphics and model demonstrations. You will also learn simple, everyday techniques for preventing strained muscles, and the important role of the foot and its arches in supporting the body in motion.

ISBN: 09629942-0-0
Paperback, 120 pages, $14.05
Packaging and postage, single book, $5.00

ABC OF ASTHMA, ALLERGIES AND LUPUS

This breakthrough scientific information uncovers the real cause of asthma, allergies and lupus. The book will serve as a guidebook for the nation's 17 million asthmatics – 14 million of them innocent children – and the 50 million who suffer from allergies. Discover why these conditions are actually your body's ways of alerting you to an urgent need for water. You'll learn how to recognize your body's true thirst signals. Discover why autoimmune diseases, such as lupus, are actually caused by unintentional dehydration. This book explains the way to treat asthma, allergies and lupus naturally, simply and at no cost. Learn the many constructive roles of salt and cholesterol in the body.

ISBN: 0-9629942-6-X
Paperback, 237 pages, $17.00
Packaging and postage, single book, $5.00

WATER: FOR HEALTH, FOR HEALING, FOR LIFE

Based on more than twenty years of clinical and scientific research into the role of water in the body, Dr. Batmanghelidj shows how water can relieve a stunning range of medical conditions. Simply adjusting your fluid and salt intakes can help you treat and prevent dozens of diseases, avoid costly prescription drugs, and enjoy vibrant new health.

Discover:
- How much water and salt you need each day to stay healthy
- Why other beverages, including tea, coffee, and sodas, cannot be substituted for water
- How to help prevent life-threatening conditions such as heart failure, stroke, Alzheimer's disease, Parkinson's disease, and cancer.
- Why water is the key to losing weight without dieting
- How to hydrate your skin to combat premature aging

ISBN – 9702458-4-X
Hard cover book, 204 pages, $17.00 (retails for $27.00)
Packaging and postage, single book, $5.00

WATER CURES: DRUGS KILL

This new book has been compiled to turn conventional medicine on its head. The revelations you'll read here will transform the practice of medicine all over the world. They will change the present cost-intensive, drug peddling, and commerce driven medical system to a physiology-based and disease preventing natural approach to health.

Water Cures: Drugs Kill contains 180 pages of case histories of people for whom the water cure worked. You will read how the conventional drug based medical system failed these people. Dr. B's observations concerning our "sick care" system, as he calls it, are not complementary!

ISBN – 0-9702458-1-5
Paperback, 228 pages, $14.95
Packaging and postage, single book, $5.00

SPECIAL REPORT: PAIN: ARTHRITIS PAIN & BACK PAIN

This special report on pain explains the importance of pain as a thirst signal of the body, and why arthritis and back pain are the same dehydration-producing signals that signify a disease-producing level of local drought in different regions of the body.

12 pages, $10.00
Packaging and postage, single report, $5.00

NEW! Spanish Edition "Your Body's Many Cries for Water"
LOS MUCHOS CLAMORES DE SU CUERPO POR AGUA
Un preventivo manual autodidáctico para los que prefieren adherirse a la lógica de lo natural y simple.

Esta es la primera edición en español del famoso libro del Dr. F.Batmaghalidj. Su mensaje ha sido recibido por millones de personas en todo el mundo, y en muchos idiomas, ahora se ha completado este sueño para él que tiene un escenario de 400 millones de almas. Se recomienda su lectura y además la adopción de sus recomendaciones. No los defraudará. El siempre dice que trabaja para Dios...nuestro creador

ISBN – 0-9702458-3-1
Paperback, 240 pages, $15.00
Packaging and postage, single book, $5.00

WATER: RX FOR A HEALTHIER, PAIN-FREE LIFE
A comprehensive handbook that also serves as a guideline to the information covered in the audio taped presentations itemized below.

For best results, read it before you listen to the tapes. It will prepare your mind so you gain maximum benefit from the information presented in the audiotape seminar. This guide is also an invaluable reference manual to recognizing your body's thirst signals...the common health problems that often result from unintentional dehydration...and how to treat them with the proper timing and correct proportions of water and salt.

50 pages, $7.00
Packaging and postage, single book, $5.00

VIDEOS & DVDs

CURE PAIN AND PREVENT CANCER
Videotaped Presentation at Yoga Research Society 1997 Conference –
Thomas Jefferson University Medical School.

Dr. Batmanghelidj explains the link between chronic pain and
cancer, and shows you how to use water and salt to relieve pain
and prevent disease in this fascinating two-hour videotaped program. In this enlightening presentation, Dr. Batmanghelidj
explains how pain is a cry from your body for more water and salt,
and is a warning sign that you could be at risk for cancer or other
serious illness. New research on how your immune system
becomes prone to uncontrolled cell overgrowth, DNA damage
and DNA repair dysfunction that leads to cancer shows a vital
dependence of your body not just on water, but on salt as well. In
fact, a whole host of d3generative diseases are linked not only to
dehydration but also to inadequate salt intake.

Dr. Batmanghelidj demonstrates why salt should be taken with
water. Learn how to use both water and salt in the proper balance. Learn why pain is a thirst signal you can't afford to ignore!
This video helps you recognize your body's emergency calls – and
easily missed silent cries – for water. Dr. Batmanghelidj presents
his latest research findings and recommendations so you'll know
exactly what steps to take to shield yourself and those close to you
from pain and disease.

ISBN: 0-9629942-9-4
2 hour, color, VHS, $30.00
Packaging and postage, single tape, $5.00

HOW TO DEAL WITH BACK PAIN

This easy-to-follow program shows you how to promote fluid circulation in your spinal discs to gain instant relief of back pain and
sciatic pain. It also exposes the latest scientific breakthroughs on

the physiology of chronic back pain. The Video provides step-by-step instructions to help you identify the source and location of your pain. It shows simple body exercises that actually normalize the position of the vertebral discs and draw the pain-causing disc away from the spinal cord to normally relieve sciatic pain within a half hour. The exercises also strengthen the "stays of your spine," back muscles, tendons and ligaments to prevent further suffering.

A safe, doctor-designed approach that has brought soothing, long-lasting comfort to thousands of viewers.

ISBN – 0-9629942-1-9
25 minutes, color, VHS, $29.95
Packaging and postage, single tape, $5.00

HEALTH MIRACLES IN WATER & SALT, CHOICE MEDICATIONS FOR CURE OF PAIN AND DISEASE, INCLUDING CANCER

Dr. B's 2-hour plus Medical Yoga 2001 lecture at Thomas Jefferson University Hospital, Department of Integrative Medicine, highlights the important disease-preventing roles of water and salt in the human body. This information represents a medical breakthrough within the science of physiology and openly challenges the sanity and sincerity of the pharmaceutical approach to the treatment of many health problems by the practitioners of conventional medicine.

ISBN 0-9702458-0-7
2 hour, color, VHS, $30.00
Packaging and postage, single tape, $5.00
(Also available as a:
DVD, $30.00, S&H, $5.00
CD set, $20.00, S&H, $5.00
Audio set, $18.00, S&H, $5.00)

NEW! DEHYDRATION AND CANCER

This video takes you to Dr. B's 2002-invited lecture at the Cancer
Control Society. In the same way the topic of the lecture stunned
the audience at the convention, this half-hour video will change
how you think about your future health. It will give you the in-
depth science behind the benefits of hydration. It will teach you
how to protect yourself from asthma, allergies and hypertension.
You will learn how to gain immediate relief from morning sickness, heartburn, and back pain. It explains how migraine
headaches, rheumatoid joint pain of fibromyalgia pain, and
indeed, all the major pains of the body denote dehydration where
you feel pain. Together, they denote ongoing complications leading to more serious disease. You will understand the roll of pH in
wellness, and discover the keys to fighting obesity, Alzheimer's,
MS and CANCER, exhaustion, depression and cravings. Learn
why, and what you can do to help yourself.

30 minutes, color, VHS, $20.00
Packaging and postage, single tape, $5.00

AUDIOTAPES & CDs

WATER: RX FOR A HEALTHIER, PAIN-FREE LIFE
*A comprehensive yet easy-to-understand, 10-hour audio course
detailing the role of water and its miraculous healing power.*

This comprehensive, 10-hour audiotape seminar gives you a firm
foundation for Dr. Batmanghelidj's natural water cure program.
You'll get answers to the most frequently asked "whys" and "hows"
of the water cure and learn how it can be used to treat a surprisingly broad range of ailments. Dr. Batman explains in detail the
body's newly discovered thirst perceptions and crisis signals of
dehydration – and why so many "disease conditions" are actually
states of dehydration that can be prevented and cured by balancing one's daily water and salt intake. These eight informative
audiotapes are ideal for anytime listening – at home, on the road

or for group discussions. They are an excellent source of information for the visually impaired.

ISBN: 0-9629942-7-8
8 tape album plus a 50-page guidebook, $67.00
8 CD album plus a 50-page guidebook, $72.00
    Packaging and postage, one album, $7.00

HEALTH MIRACLES IN WATER & SALT, CHOICE MEDICATIONS
    FOR CURE OF PAIN AND DISEASE, INCLUDING CANCER
    See explanation of lecture listed under Videos and DVDs

CD set, $20.00, S&H $5.00
Audio set $18.00, S&H $5.00

YOUR BODY'S MANY CRIES FOR WATER
Lecture at the 39th PA Annual Natural Living Conference
at Kutztown University, Kutztown, PA 1993

The lecture got a standing ovation! Learn where and when the water cure was discovered. Learn the way Alexander Fleming discovered penicillin. Learn what he told Dr. Batmanghelidj when he was Sir Alexander's student. Learn why water can permanently erase pain and counteract the effects of stress. Discover the pain-relieving properties of water and why pain is a sign of serious, system-wide dehydration. Learn how you can shut off pain without aspirin, NSAIDS and other side-effect-ridden drugs. You'll be inspired by the real-life examples of people who have used the "watercure" to put an end to their pain and suffering.

90 minutes, $10.00
Packaging and postage, single tape, $3.00

Water: The New Immune Breakthrough & Pain and Cancer
"Wonder Drug" Capital University of Integrative Medicine: Postgraduate Guest Lecture Tape

In this tape/CD, you will hear what a group of postgraduate health care professionals, including medical doctors and chiropractors, learned about dehydration as the primary cause of the painful degenerative diseases of the human body. This tape/CD contains information on how cancer occurs when there is long-term shortage of water in the body. Two case histories of breast cancer and lymphoma that have gone into remission because of increased water intake are introduced.

95 minutes, $10.00; packaging and postage, single tape, $3.00
CD set, $18.00; packaging and postage, $5.00

Water & Salt: Rx for Total Healing
Tape of Dr. F. Batmanghelidj's opening address at 1999 Pennsylvania Annual Natural Living Conference, Cedar Crest College Allentown, PA

Learn the many health benefits of taking sea salt when you are drinking adequate water. Dr. B will explain the need for salt and the dangers of a salt free diet. He will address the challenges of hypertension and explain the damage done by diuretics.

90 minutes, $10.00
Packaging and postage, single tape, $3.00

Multiple Sclerosis: Is "Water" Its Cure?
Real-life Evidence of the Link between Dehydration and MS

In this lively audiotape of the "Just Common Sense" radio program hosted by Bob Butts, you will hear from a young male MS sufferer who used Dr. Batman's water and salt program to put an end to his symptoms. This revealing interview with Dr. Batman explains how you can use the same water and salt cure to bring relief to the incapacitating fatigue, swelling and vision and cognitive problems that plague MS sufferers. He also discusses the destructive effects of caffeine on memory and energy.

69 minutes, $10.00
Packaging and postage, single tape, $3.00

To order the above items, send check or money order to:

Global Health Solutions
2146 King's Garden Way
Falls Church, VA 22043, USA
Tel. 703-848-2333 10:00am -6:00pm EST
Fax: 703-848-0028

Discount given for orders of five or more books
VISA, MasterCard and Discover orders only:
1-800-759-3999

VA state tax should be added to orders by Virginia residents

Or order on our website:
Website address: www.watercure.com